A PLUME BOOK

THE BLACK BOOK OF HOLLYWOOD BEAUTY SECRETS

KYM DOUGLAS is a beauty and fashion correspondent for *The View*, and is the host of Lifetime's new makeover series *Queen*. She also appears on *Soap Talk, Good Day L.A., Before and Afternoon's*, and *Your Weekend with Jim Brickman*. She lives in Encino, California, with her husband of twenty-one years; their eight-year-old son, Hunter; a 110-pound golden retriever, Gatsby; and a hamster named Waffle.

CINDY PEARLMAN is a nationally syndicated writer for the *New York Times* syndicate and the *Chicago Sun-Times*. She's written many books, including *You Gotta See This* (Plume) and, coauthored with model Janice Dickinson, the bestselling beauty and dating book *Everything About Me Is Fake . . . and I'm Perfect*. Cindy's work has appeared frequently in *Entertainment Weekly, People, Self, InTouch, National Geographic, Ladies Home Journal, Redbook*, and *Seventeen*. Cindy lives in the suburbs of Chicago with her two large dogs, Jake and Cody. They don't care if she has about three million beauty products in the bathroom.

You can reach Kym and Cindy and learn the latest beauty secrets at www.blackbookbeautysecrets.com.

Tips from . . .

Scarlett Johansson, Jennifer Aniston,
Charlize Theron, Catherine Zeta-Jones,
Paris Hilton, Lindsay Lohan,
Queen Latifah, Evan Rachel Wood,
Jessica Simpson, Sheryl Crow,
Alexis Bledel, Kelly Ripa,
Cindy Crawford, Julianne Moore,
Salma Hayek, Heather Graham,
Hilary Swank, Elizabeth Hurley,
Jennifer Lopez, Amber Valletta,
Naomi Watts, Sienna Miller,
Mariah Carey, Cameron Diaz,
Jennifer Garner, Beyoncé Knowles,

And more . . .

The Black Book of
Hollywood
Beauty
Secrets

Kym Douglas
and Cindy Pearlman

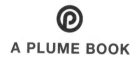

A PLUME BOOK

PLUME
Published by Penguin Group
Penguin Group (USA) Inc., 375 Hudson Street, New York, New York 10014, U.S.A.
Penguin Group (Canada), 90 Eglinton Avenue East, Suite 700, Toronto, Ontario, Canada
M4P 2Y3 (a division of Pearson Penguin Canada Inc.)
Penguin Books Ltd., 80 Strand, London WC2R 0RL, England
Penguin Ireland, 25 St. Stephen's Green, Dublin 2, Ireland (a division of Penguin Books Ltd.)
Penguin Group (Australia), 250 Camberwell Road, Camberwell, Victoria 3124, Australia
(a division of Pearson Australia Group Pty. Ltd.)
Penguin Books India Pvt. Ltd., 11 Community Centre, Panchsheel Park,
New Delhi – 110 017, India
Penguin Books (NZ), cnr Airborne and Rosedale Roads, Albany, Auckland 1310,
New Zealand (a division of Pearson New Zealand Ltd.)
Penguin Books (South Africa) (Pty.) Ltd., 24 Sturdee Avenue, Rosebank, Johannesburg 2196,
South Africa

Penguin Books Ltd., Registered Offices: 80 Strand, London WC2R 0RL, England

First published by Plume, a member of Penguin Group (USA) Inc.

First Printing, December 2006
10   9   8   7   6   5   4   3   2   1

 REGISTERED TRADEMARK—MARCA REGISTRADA

LIBRARY OF CONGRESS CATALOGING-IN-PUBLICATION DATA

Douglas, Kym.
    The black book of hollywood beauty secrets : by Kym Douglas and Cindy Pearlman.
       p.   cm.
    ISBN 0-452-28765-0
       1. Beauty, Personal.   2. Cosmetics.   3. Motion picture actors and actresses—Health and
hygiene.   I. Pearlman, Cindy, 1964–   II.   Title.
    RA778.D738   2006
    646.7'042—dc22

                                                                                2006015388

Printed in the United States of America
Set in Esprit Book

FROM KYM:

To my mother and father, Barbara and
John Bankier, who give me unwavering love,
nurturing, and encouragement
every day of my life.

To my husband of twenty-one years,
Jerry Douglas, who has always followed his
heart and soul and helped me to follow mine.

To my eight-year-old son, Hunter William
Douglas, you are all that is beautiful, loving,
and kind . . . you are my gift from God.

FROM CINDY:

To my mother and father, Renee and Paul
Pearlman, who gave me love, spirit, and faith
in myself and insisted that I follow my dreams.

To Michael Drapp, who teaches me daily about
the most beautiful part of life, which is true
love and the meaning of Being One.

LOVE. FAMILY. DREAMS.

**THEY'RE THE BIGGEST BEAUTY
SECRETS OF ALL.**

Life isn't about finding yourself; life is
about creating yourself.
—**George Bernard Shaw**

Who am I to judge anybody? I had bangs in the '80s.
—**Sarah Jessica Parker**

CONTENTS

INTRODUCTION

Once Upon an Uglier Time . . .

Cheerleaders.

It's all their fault.

Every Friday in the Midwest, we sat in the back of the class with the other rejects watching "them"—pretty, skinny, tall, straight- and shiny-haired, freakin' cheerleaders, aka "them"—bounce into homeroom in their crisp, leg-flashing miniskirts and school-color-blazing, boob-defining sweaters.

Even their breasts screamed, "I belong" in unison like a tiny, C-cup popularity cheer.

There sat the rest of us wishing, hoping, praying the same mantra over and over again: "Why can't that be me?"

Why not? We didn't have the skin, the hair, the bodies, the height, or the boobs. We didn't even own school sweaters. Instead we had low self-esteem, acne, and free weekends.

We still had our dreams. Fast-forward a decade to see Kym leaving Detroit and Cindy commuting to Hollywood weekly because now the two most normal, former dorks on the planet had been magically plucked from obscurity to become entertainment reporters covering the Hollywood beat for network television and major newspapers. (Can you even believe it?)

Suddenly, two frizzy-haired girls from the Heartland had glamorous careers that had us rubbing shoulders with the world's most beautiful, sexy, successful people for major television shows including *The View* and *Good Day L.A.*, and leading newspapers such as the *New York Times* and *Chicago Sun-Times*. We were roaming the streets of Los Angeles and Beverly Hills where we learned a startling secret, painful to reveal: Hollywood is . . . a lot like high school except EVERYONE is a cheerleader.

Again, we didn't have the skin, the hair, the bodies, the height, or those big, artificial boobs. We could afford new TSE cashmere sweaters, but now it wasn't about ancient school colors. It was about wearing the right letters of high-end designers—RL, Gucci, Prada, Fendi, Louie, D&G, Chanel, etc. Did we really have to wear the word "Juicy" over our derrieres to get a reservation at Koi, the hottest restaurant in Beverly Hills (Translation: the cool table in the school cafeteria)?

The questions didn't end there. Why did we see fine lines forming, along with pimples. Why did all those actresses over 30 feel the right to bare arms even though, as good Americans, we know that it's clearly stated in the Constitution that this is illegal. (Meanwhile, our naked arms haven't experienced fresh air since the late '70s.)

How in the name of all that is good and fat free could Demi Moore at age 40 wear a bikini and a full-length mink coat on the big screen and not look fat, while at the same time dating and then marrying a 12-year-old? She wasn't even a cheerleader in our eyes, but something far worse. She was the freakin' homecoming queen of Beverly Hills.

Would we ever graduate from this beauty nightmare?

*   *   *

Our solution was to become students of beauty and approach the topic with the drive and precision of Harvard biomedical researchers. Ours were the most perfect specimens on earth: Uma Thurman with the porcelain, poreless skin, and Jennifer Aniston with the stick-straight, frizz-free, ultrashiny hair, even through the divorce and the relocation to humid Malibu. There was the amazonically wonderful Nicole Kidman, the seriously rounded, booty-shaking Beyoncé—or was it J.Lo (they're interchangeable when it comes to their backsides)—and the bubbly, naturally big-boobed Jessica Simpson. Let's just elect her as our squad leader.

In our day jobs, we had ample opportunity to dissect "the popular girls of Hollywood." To our utter dismay, they weren't even bitchy. We examined, analyzed, investigated, inspected, and scrutinized everything "they" did to look so perfect. When that got too complicated, we dropped the Jane Bond act and just asked them how they did it. What did they use? How often did they use it? Where did they get it? How much did it cost? How can we do it, too?

And they told us.

We couldn't believe it either.

There were too many amazing tips to remember, so we wrote them down.

And so, *The Black Book of Hollywood Beauty Secrets* was born.

Are you in or are you out?

For years, we've followed the advice of these Hollywood women and seen our skin, our bods, and our hair magically transformed. Of course, we didn't get picked to join beauty pageants and directors didn't cast us in big-budget movies. Yet, people began to ask, "What the heck are you doing right?"

When Kim Basinger told us to use scuba-diver oil on our faces, we stocked up. (It worked wonders, and the guys in the scuba store were darn cute.)

When Teri Hatcher told us to bathe in red wine to soften our skin, we got out two glasses and filled our respective tubs. Hello, she didn't say you needed to use the entire bottle in the tub. (Teri is obviously the fun cheerleader!)

We even stopped saying the following words on a daily basis: "If only we could have Jennifer Aniston's hair, Jessica Simpson's body, Gwyneth Paltrow's flawless skin, and Catherine Zeta-Jones's cheekbones, our lives would be fabulous and Brad Pitt would magically appear with a bottle of really expensive red wine and some fabulous takeout sushi." Of course save some wine for the bath.

We had to stop saying all of the above because it's a lot of words and Brad is technically a taken man, Kym is married, and Cindy has a boyfriend.

But we digress. Some of the advice we culled from the celebrities themselves and some from their top advisors— their makeup artists, style gurus, and hair people. Of course, some of it seemed just a little bit too much. We love Lisa Rinna, but we can't rub male foreskin lotion on . . . anything. Honestly, we also couldn't rub cow placenta on our faces as a moisturizer. It was just a little too gross and the last thing we needed was a call from PETA asking us to give those cows back their personal parts.

Too stressful. And Susan Sarandon warned us, "Ladies,

stress shows up on your face. Happiness is the true beauty weapon." And who were we to disagree with someone who still wears deep-V-neck Armani dresses held up by real cleavage? At this point in the game the V-neck dress is better than a too-tight letterman sweater. Just ask **Tim Robbins**.

What follows in these pages is the best of the best tips we learned. They're simple, often inexpensive, ways to boost your beauty IQ given to us by people who make their living by looking their best.

In the end, the best thing we learned didn't come from any celebrity. It came from turning 40 and realizing that we were luckier than teenage girls. Who really wanted to peak at age 17 and just be the girl rah-rahing for someone else?

We even had to accept our bodies, the good and the bad, the positive and the negative, and just say, "Yeah, me!" We try to say it often while not looking at our thighs, which are still much too big, if you ask us.

The other day, Kym even said, "Hey, maybe now we're ready for cheerleading tryouts."

Cindy replied, "But we might only make alternates."

Kym sighed and said, "God, isn't that enough."

CHAPTER 1

Roll Out the Red Carpet: A Pre-Primping Primer

Hollywood has its own lingo, which cannot be ignored in covering the beauty industry. In order for you to talk the talk, we'd like to present what we'll call HOLLYWOOD BEAUTY SPEAK. Think of this as a primer for beauty understanding. Please read this in the proper light. Don't squint and thus form fine lines—*the horror, the horror!*

XO,
Kym and Cindy

HOLLYWOOD BEAUTY SPEAK

RENEWAL: Instead of saying you're having a face-lift or a shot of Botox, say, "I'm sorry **Demi**, but I can't meet you at the Ivy for chopped salads tomorrow because I'm going in for a renewal." Her response should be something like, "Oh, I understand. I had a renewal last week."

BOTOXIC: A woman who has had so much Botox that she doesn't have an expression left in her, but she still tells her girlfriends that they should get shot up. For example: "Don't listen to her about your forehead. She's Botoxic."

BRITNEY-ITIS: If you don't immediately drop all of your weight in the hospital before you bring your baby home, you're experiencing Britney-itis. Get out the tunic tops and the roomy sweats; e.g., "Poor Angie. Did you see her at Trader Joe's? Little Shiloh is adorable, but Angie has a bad case of Britney-itis."

BFF (BEST FRIEND FOREVER): The equivalent of your grown-up best friend in Hollywood or Beverly Hills, but with a twist. You're sharing the Shu Uemura products today and hating each other's well-toned guts the next. BFF is not lasting. Think Paris and Nicole. Think Cindy and George Clooney, or Kym and Nicole Kidman. Wait, those last two were just dream BFFs.

NEW BEST FRIENDS: Known her for years, never spoken to her. Might even include air kissing when you see her at the salon or spa.

FOREVER GETTING READY FOR THE PROM: How women past 25 feel during their hour-plus hair and makeup regime to go on a date, to the office, or even to Walgreens to get the latest issue of *InStyle*. Translation: "I know I've been in the bathroom since morning. What can I do? I'm forever getting ready for the prom."

IT'S NOT LISTED: A new, good, A-lister's, insider's restaurant or beauty salon that's not listed in the phone book, has no address, and has no sign out front. For example, "Hey, Keira is in from England. Want to go to that place on Wilshire. It's not listed."

IT BAG: There is no need to call a Fendi a purse. Heaven forbid! It's an It Bag.

GETTING MY WIG BLOWN OUT: Going to the hair salon to get your real hair done for an event.

PAPARAZZI READY: Looking and feeling really good. As in, "Yes, you can send the limo right now because I'm paparazzi ready."

PULLING AN OLSEN: A nicer way to say that you're doing an extreme low-carb diet in order to fit into your sleekest Calvin Klein summer dress. To your Hollywood executive husband: "You can eat pizza with the kids tonight, but I'll have salad because I'm pulling an Olsen."

FULLY LANDSCAPED: Used to describe someone who doesn't have hair in places where she doesn't want hair. As in, "Yes, I saw her at Canyon Ranch Spa the other day and she was fully landscaped."

TROPICAL MOMENT: Peri- or post-menopausal hot flashes or night sweats. For example: You're at the Grammys in the middle of winter and Cher looks flushed. You say: "Are you all right?" Cher: "Oh, yes, I'm just having a tropical moment."

HE'S SO YOGA: Someone who is so flexible and in such great shape that it's obvious he must be doing yoga. For example, "I wish my husband could look like Sting. He's just so yoga. [Pause] No, I don't mean my husband."

SHE'S SPONGE: A Hollywood girl who doesn't share her info about hair, nails, or good prices on clothes. She's just about who YOU go to and where YOU got your stuff. All the moms at the private schools will pick one woman out and say, "Don't talk to her. She's sponge."

WE'RE IN THE MIDDLE OF A PARIS AND NICOLE RIGHT NOW: This is for when you have a serious tiff with your BFF (best friend forever). Example: "Where is Amber? I thought she was meeting us at the Gardens restaurant at the Four Seasons for lobster clubs?" Answer: "She won't be coming. We're in the middle of a Paris and Nicole." It's like an adult time-out. There is no Hollywood Supernanny to offer a cure.

STEP AWAY FROM THE KRISPY KREMES: A nice way to tell a friend that she needs to drop a few pounds.

THICK SKIN: Skin that looks good without any plastic surgery (yet); e.g., "Do you think she's had anything done? No, I'm pretty sure it's natural. We hate her. It's thick skin."

YOUR NEW LOOK IS WAITING. BUT FIRST, A FEW WORDS FROM YOUR BEAUTY SPONSORS

The Black Book of Hollywood Beauty Secrets rips back that red carpet and rolls the limo back to the stars' homes. It's a timeless beauty reference book that invites you into the bathrooms and medicine cabinets of the biggest A-list celebs on the planet, as well as their makeup artists. We'll show you how you can look and feel just as fabulous as they do.

Now, it's time to get to the tips.

GLAMMING UP

Hollywood's Secret Number One: Remember that most celebrities are cheapskates. If they don't get it for free, they won't use it. Since even they don't get everything for free, most celebs rely on inexpensive, organic, yes, even cheap, natural beauty tricks.

Hollywood's Secret Number Two: Forget about the extreme makeover. One or two tiny changes can revamp your entire look. With the tips in this book, you can make simple changes that will kiss your "before" days good-bye—forever!

We can't promise you any one of the **Jennifers'** lives (**Aniston**, **Garner**, or **Lopez**—and why are there so many Jennifers anyway, we ask?). We can promise to reveal the ways they fight zits, give great face, and work out before a premiere.

We're going to start with the face and work our way down the beauty trail with chapters about skin care, makeup secrets, hair solutions, body-shaping tips, and accessorizing how-to's. We'll give you a two-weeks-to-the-big-event glam crash course and even a stripper secret about always looking perky.

Happy makeovers, kittens.

While you get ready for your close-up, we'll throw in a bit of celebrity beauty gossip. (We all need a little inside dish just to divert ourselves from the fact that our Manolos are killing us.)

Overheard on the Red Carpet: What wild Hollywood tart has so many shoes that when she travels to Europe she gets a room for herself and a room for her shoes? Yes, Miss Thing recently stayed in a $4,000-a-night room in Paris and her shoes stayed next door in an equally pricey suite. No word if the shoes ordered room service or "accidentally" went home with the plush robe.

CHAPTER 2

Skin: Face Your Fans

My makeup artist tells me my face is the size of a bus.
—**Charlize Theron**

Sleep is the biggest beauty secret of all. What kind of girl goes to bed at 8:30 P.M.? In my case a happy one.
—**Catherine Zeta-Jones**, who mentions that husband
Michael Douglas is also a pretty happy guy

We're dangerously close to an age of nirvana when women and men can celebrate world peace while injecting Crème de la Mer intravenously without lifting a flawlessly manicured finger to touch up roots via satellite laser beam. Dare to dream. Back in the real world where we only pray for such beauty heaven, most of us either sleep in our socks and mascara or spend a good forty-five minutes in the bathroom completing the Olympics of skin-care regimes. Put down that generic moisturizer, drop the scrub, stop fretting over your under-eye bags, and read on for some truly spectacular celeb skin-care secrets that will make you look as flawless as **Nicole** or **Angelina**.

SHINY AND THE CITY

Sarah Jessica Parker, who was recently named one of the wealthiest women in New York, has a beauty secret that anyone can afford. The former *Sex and the City* siren says that despite being financially solid, she still likes to save a penny or two when possible, especially since she grew up helping to support her large family with her acting jobs. We think she's perfect, but allegedly even **Sarah** gets a little oily in her T-zone (chin, nose, and forehead). When you feel a little shine in those areas, do as **SJP** does: Politely excuse yourself to the ladies' room and pull out one of those tissue toilet-seat covers from the wall of the bathroom stall. Don't sit on it, silly. Tear off a small piece of the seat cover and dab it on your chin, nose, and forehead. The tissue is so soft and lightweight it perfectly absorbs facial oil and keeps your makeup in place. You just saved yourself about $25 because pricey designer blotting pads do exactly the same thing.

BB Extra: The tissue paper pricier stores wrap your new Calvin Klein silk undies in also works as a fabulous blotter.

GIVING GOOD FACE: JENNIFER ANISTON

Because she is one of our favorite beauty role models and because she might have killed us if we focused on her notorious hair, we asked **Jennifer Aniston** what in the world she does to keep her famous puss looking so clear and line-free. (**Jen** was so shocked we left her locks out of it, she couldn't wait to answer.) No, it wasn't all those mascara-stained tissues after Brad that moisturized her skin. It was cheap soap! "You're going to hate me for this, but I don't go out and buy only the expensive stuff," Jennifer confided. "Most nights, I just wash my face with Neutrogena facial soap."

And while we're on the topic of her epidermis, Jen took another sip of tea over breakfast at the Ritz-Carlton in Pasadena and revealed her other cheapo beauty fave, which costs a lot less than the $75 egg whites on her plate. "I love the lavender body scrub that they sell at Trader Joe's. It's only six dollars and really fabulous."

SUCKING UP, SCRUBBING OFF

Top Los Angeles skin-care guru Heather Hale—who just gave Kym a fabulous two-hour facial called the Skin Master, exclusive to Dr. Patrick Abergel's Institute in tawny Santa Monica, California—says you don't have to go to that big store in the mall named after an Egyptian goddess for exfoliating sponges. "This is actually a beauty tip given to me by my mom. I keep a kitchen sponge in my shower," Heather tells us. "You know, the one that is yellow and spongy on one side and rough and green on the other." You don't need a user's manual to figure it out. "While in the shower I suds up the rough green side and use it to cleanse and exfoliate the bottoms of my feet. It exfoliates just as well as any foot file and it is a lot easier to use!" By the way, you can buy these sponges in bulk at Costco. And do toss them so they don't grow any weird green things inside.

Overheard on the Red Carpet: We know this major A-list TV star shuns chocolate—too many calories. But she has a strange habit of wrapping her entire body in it. She travels to a chichi Texas spa where she gets a sixty-minute heat-sealing chocolate paraffin body wrap. She's coddled in cocoa powder and raspberry chocolate truffle oil. She even gets the twenty-minute chocolate massage, mud mask, and a large piece of chocolate cake to finish the process. (She never eats the cake.)

A Very Sticky Situation

We hate to take away business from any major skin-care line. So, keep this one quiet, but give it a try. Ditch those sticky pads that you use to rid your nose and T-zone of blackheads. Legally, we can't mention them here, but you know what they are. Instead, smear a thin strip of Elmer's Glue onto your T-zone, or what we'll call Clog Land. Let it dry and then gently peel it off. (Remember doing this as a kid and pouring the glue all over your hands? It's just as fun now.) It's also a cheap alternative that actually works. And when you're finished, you can take the rest of the bottle and help your kids with their school art projects.

FOOD FOR FACE—PART ONE

Let's take a quick chauffeured Bentley ride through the ways you can cure your most common skin problems with foods you can whip up in a jiffy—even if your name is not **Rachael Ray.**

- Eat your bruschetta. Toast with tomatoes and olive oil contains antiaging fighters that stop collagen from breaking down by 35 percent.

- Sweet potatoes are a sweet deal for your sparkling eyes. Those tasty treats are rich in carotenoids and these act as natural sunglasses, blocking out damaging UV lights. Also, the lutein found in sweet potatoes stops the damage of aging and can actually make your vision clearer.

- Pomegranate juice does contain natural antioxidants. If you drink it daily you'll see fine lines start to vanish.

- Bananas also help rid you of wrinkles. Mash one-fourth of a banana until creamy and spread on your face. Leave on for twenty minutes, rinse off with warm water, then dash on cold. Your pores will feel very tight, and your face will smell yummy.

CELE-BEAUTY: LISA RINNA

A Note from Kym: I met Lisa Rinna about twenty years ago when she was a struggling actress dating a gorgeous young actor named Peter Barton who was on my husband's show, *The Young and the Restless*. She was a fresh-faced brunette beauty with a gregarious laugh and a tenacious drive to succeed that was unmatched by anyone I've ever met. Succeed she did! She starred on *Days of Our Lives*, *Melrose Place*, and *Dancing with the Stars*, and hosts the Emmy-nominated *Soap Talk*. Lisa is also a boutique owner, designer, now wife of handsome hunk Harry Hamlin, and the mother of two daughters.

The thing that has always stuck with me about Lisa was an interview I did with her when I was a fresh entertainment reporter on E! Entertainment Television. I would routinely ask the starlets how they got and kept such fabulous figures. Lisa was on *Melrose Place* at the time. All the other actresses answered the question with, "Gosh I don't know, I eat whatever I want and I never work out. I guess I just have a fast metabolism. Blah blah blah."

Lisa said in a proud, strong voice, "How do I keep my body like this? I work my ass off."

Okay, let's cut to the chase. While we're interested in all of Lisa's answers, what we really want to know is what she uses on her luscious lips—and can we use it, too? It's MAC Prrr lip gloss.

Now read on for her other secrets . . .

What is a high-end, over-the-top expensive, just-can't-live-without purchase for beauty?
Epicuren Orange Blossom body cream.

What is your favorite inexpensive or homemade beauty tip or product?
Egg-white masks for tightening my pores.

What are your all-time, never-fail, top-five best beauty products that you can't live without?
ChapStick. The black one. Original. Aquaphor from the drugstore for chapped skin, MAC Prrr lip gloss, Lorac Mommy Kit makeup palette, Nars Ginger concealer.

If you were going to your own private island and could take only one skin-care product, what would it be?

ChapStick.

What is your secret antiaging tip?

Mario Badescu lifting mask.

What sets a starlet, socialite, or true beauty apart from all the other girls in the pack?

A lot more maintence work has to be done. I call it **"Forever getting ready for the prom."**

Give us your favorite health and diet tip (besides drinking water).

Food combining!

What do you do a month before, a week before, and the day of a big event to make sure you look your very best?

For a big event a month out, I do nothing different. A week out, I cut down on my starches and carbs. Get a bikini wax, exercise a bit more with harder workouts, then a self-tan and my hair cut and colored. The day of the big event, I hang with my family, low-key, do yoga, eat a nice breakfast and lunch and have my favorite hair and makeup team (Faye Woods and Adam Christopher) come to my house to get me ready. I feel really safe with them and they are The Best. We laugh and that's the best thing you can do to look good for your big event!

What is the most common beauty blunder?
Too much blush!

Who would you most like to have dinner with to discuss her beauty tips?
Patricia Wexler (she is a top NYC dermatologist to the stars).

What is the craziest, wackiest thing you have ever done or tried for beauty?
Everything is for maintenance and it's all crazy. I do photo facials, microdermabrasion, peels, regular facials, etc., etc.

Please tell us one secret beauty tip that you share only with your closest friends.
I share all my beauty tips with my friends. My biggest tip is Dr. Harold Lancer in Beverly Hills, California. He is one of the top dermatologists in the country and Kym Douglas goes to him, too! [NOTE: Dr. Harold Lancer has been my own personal dermatologist for over twenty years. He is a magician with skin and makes all the starlets in town look fabulous for the red carpet. He is a perfectionist and has his own line of skin care called The Glow! He will not tell you this, but I have bumped into Madonna in his valet parking, Diane Lane on the elevator, Lisa Marie Presley in his hallway, and Beyoncé . . . just to name a few of his "I won't name" clients. He's the best. I love you Dr. Lancer! And can you get me in for my next appointment before 2008?]

What toothpaste do you use, conditioner, shampoo, perfume, favorite designer, jeans? . . .

Perfume none, I'm allergic. Toothpaste, any baking soda–peroxide one. Shampoo/conditioner Kérastase, the yellow ones. Jeans—I like J Brand and True Religion.

What is your favorite at-home, in-a-quick-pinch home remedy for beautiful skin or hair?
I just take a quick shower. Fresh always looks good.

Give us the most unusual, unique, out-of-the-ordinary item you have ever used on yourself or someone else to make them look more beautiful.
I once used this product that has men's foreskin in it! Yikes!

Overheard on the Red Carpet: What porcelain-skinned flawless beauty and A-lister likes to multitask when it comes to beauty? She requested as many as eight estheticians to work on her at the same time at a certain five-star spa. Miss Oscar nominee believes in hands-on face-buffing, moisturizing, skin-whitening, pore-refining, Swedish deep-tissue massage, and a pedicure and manicure all at the same time. The only thing she doesn't have time for is finding a new man.

FOOD FOR FACE—PART TWO: OLD-FASHIONED OATS

Oatmeal is not just good for cold winter mornings. It's a great way to reduce redness and improve your complexion. Try this all-natural beauty recipe: Mix old-fashioned oats with water to form a paste, apply to your face, and leave it on for fifteen minutes.

IMAGE MAKER: SONYA DAKAR

Call them the Dakar driven. Gwyneth, Drew, Britney, LeAnn, and Amber refuse to live without her. Gwyneth even sends for her products from across the pond. She's top facialist to the stars, Sonya Dakar. Drew Barrymore also uses the products and enthuses, "I don't know what I'd do without Sonya. Her zit cream is the only one that works. I run to her at all costs."

What does Sonya think? We put down our makeup sponges for a second and asked her.

What are your five favorite products in your bathroom right now?

- *Fresh Eyes*. This is a hydrating eye cleanser made with wheat germ and carrot-seed oil. I use it to cleanse my eye area and sometimes even my face.

- *Visualift Eye Cream*. It's the best eye cream I've ever tried. It actually helps with dark circles and fine lines—fast!

- *Cellular Patch Cream*. It's the ultimate in antiaging, plus it firms and plumps my skin.

- *Omega-3 Repair Complex*. Complex made with botanical flaxseed oil. It calms my skin and nourishes it from the inside out.

- **365 SPF30**. I avoid the sun so this is a definite must.

If you only had $100 to spend on products, what would you buy?

That is a hard one. I believe that skin care is more important than nice clothes, hair, or makeup. Your face is your business card, and it never goes out of style—it is the best investment you can make in yourself. But if I had only $100 I would buy a Mini-Kit for Irritation (it has six deluxe-size products) and then add my Visualift Eye Cream.

What is your best antiaging tip?

Avoid the sun. And never skip your nightly skin regimen.

What was your biggest beauty blunder?

I overprocessed my skin. People want results and they overdo it to their skin. Overprocessed skin can lead to premature aging, overly sensitive skin, and rosacea.

What is one secret beauty tip that you share only with your closest friends?

Use your facial products on your neck, chest, and hands. Your face is not the only place that is affected by aging, acne, discoloration, or other skin problems.

What is your favorite in-a-quick-pinch home-beauty remedy?

I do a quick mini-facial. I exfoliate with my Enzyme Peeling Cream and follow with a soft hydrating Blue Mask. After that I apply enormous amounts of moisturizer and eye cream. I especially put on a generous amount of product before I go to bed.

RECIPES FOR RIGHTEOUS BEAUTY

Just in case you're busy at a premiere on the other coast or working the school bake sale, we asked Sonya to offer some home alternatives that can add luster to your looks. Thanks, Sonya!

Celebrity Favorite Product from Sonya: Drying Potion, $25
Home Recipe Alternative:

Sonya Dakar's Secret "Zit Zapper"

GET IT:
  1 package of dry yeast
  Water

MIX IT: Pour yeast into a bowl and add water (one drop at a time), mixing well after each drop, until this mixture becomes a medium paste.

DO IT: Dot this mixture on breakouts (may be used for body breakouts, too!). Allow to dry (about thirty seconds) before hopping into bed.

WHY, WHY, WHY: Yeast will kill bacteria and dry out breakouts.

Celebrity Favorite Product: Green Tea Mask, $65

Home Recipe Alternative:

Creamy Green Tea Mask

GET IT:

    1 tea bag of green tea
    2 tablespoons of sour cream
    1 egg yolk
    1 teaspoon of olive oil
    1 teaspoon honey

MIX IT: Boil the green tea bag in ¼ cup of water until it has boiled down to 1 tablespoon, then cool in the fridge for 15 minutes. Mix all other ingredients for about 30–60 seconds, until well blended. Stir in the cooled green tea concentrate. Spread mixture over cleansed and exfoliated skin and leave on for about 15 minutes. Note: This is a soft mask and will not dry.

DO IT: Rinse well with warm water and follow with a natural toner, moisturizer, etc.

WHY, WHY, WHY?: With ingredients like soothing green tea, cooling sour cream, hydrating olive oil, and nourishing egg yolk, your sensitive skin will never be the same. Green tea is full of antioxidants and calming properties. Sour cream has lipids and proteins to soothe and nourish dry, sensitive skin and make it silky. Honey has been used as a beauty product since the days of Cleopatra. It is a natural humectant, which means it has the ability to attract and retain moisture. The skin's ability to stay moist (or hydrated) is an important factor in its ability to maintain softness and elasticity. As skin ages, or as it isexposed to environmental stresses and chemical agents, it loses this ability and grows dry and appears wrinkled. Because it's all natural and doesn't irritate the skin, honey is also suitable for sensitive skin. Egg yolk's concentrated fat and protein is incredibly nourishing. Olive oil, full of vitamins, minerals, and proteins, is gentle on sensitive skin and attracts moisture and holds it close to the skin. It forms a breathable film to prevent moisture loss and won't clog pores.

Celebrity Favorite Product from Sonya: Puffiness/Puffy Eyes
Visualift Eye Cream $105
Home Recipe Alternative:

Tea for You

GET IT:
    2 potato slices
    Chamomile tea
    Aloe vera gel

Mix it: Slice one small piece off of a potato; soak in chamomile tea, and dip in aloe vera gel.

Do it: Put one slice under each eye and leave them there for 20 minutes.

Why, why, why?: Potatoes are rich with alpha lipoic acids and safe enough to use under eyes to calm inflammation and help lighten circles. Aloe vera is a natural moisturizer, healer, and skin soother that will help tighten and reduce puffiness. People have been drinking chamomile tea for centuries because of its calming properties, but did you know it has a similar, soothing effect when used on the skin? The use of chamomile dates back 2,000 years to ancient Egypt, where women crushed the petals of the flower to beautify and protect their skin from harsh, dry weather.

IMAGE MAKER: RASHEL POURI

Rashel Pouri gives them good face, and "them" includes Vivica A. Fox, Traci Bingham, and Kelly Clarkson—and those are just the babes she can mention. Rashel, who runs Medi-Spa and Ravi Skin Care, told us that she wants all women to face the facts before they go red-carpet wrangling. "You have to take care of your skin. It's your number one job when it comes to a daily routine," says the woman whose Night Rejuvenate whole body cream has been used by Jennifer Lopez. (In fact, J.Lo's father has stocked up on it in order to bring the goods to his daughter. Come on! How many dads get their daughters night cream? A new wrinkle on being a concerned parent!)

As for Rashel, a former model who has been helping with reconstructive surgery efforts for those disfigured in Iraq, well, she provided us with a few of her best beauty tips.

- "The first step, ladies, is to keep your hands off your face during the day. Stop rubbing your cheeks. Be gentle with that skin."

- "I find it helpful to look back to my grandmother's ways, which included using a lot of fruit. You should eat fruit and also put it on your face. Both ways give you the natural vitamins you need to feed your skin."

- "This must be set in stone. No matter how much you party, you must come home and take your makeup off. If you don't take your makeup off you close the pores at night and your skin will not be able to breathe while you sleep. Remember that when you're sleeping, your skin is also supposed to be resting. It can't rest if it is covered in makeup."

- "Water, water, water. Drink a lot of water. It's key to great skin."

- "Get a clarifying facial once a month. The rest of your regime should include cleanser, toner, and moisturizer. If you're over 35, I also recommend microdermabrasian. Over-35 skin also needs night cream and eye cream, although I began using both of those when I was 19 and have never regretted it."

● "Consider a photo facial because you'll see the results right away. It's done with a laser and is not painful or uncomfortable. It begins with a thick gel on your skin and then a laser gun on your face. The procedure takes about twenty or thirty minutes and all the celebrities do it at lunchtime. It costs around $399. It gets rid of fine lines, freckles, and sun spots. A lot of people also have broken capillaries and it can get rid of those, too."

● "For the rest of the skin on my body, I do a sugar scrub. It gives you the skin of a baby."

● "Remember not to get stuck in that over-40 Botox rush. The women want collagen and botox to the point where they end up looking abnormal or like a statue. They become obsessed. My husband has said to me, 'Please honey, don't. I like a natural look.'"

FACIAL SMOOTHIES

How can you get your three servings of fruit and avoid a gargantuan carbohydrate intake for the day? Well, you can use fruit (and veggies) on your face. Rashel Pouri was happy to give us a few of her favorite facial smoothies that have amazing results:

● Want to look like you just had a collagen injection without actually paying for it? Go to your local produce aisle. "Take a peach, cut the meat off of it, and smoosh it into a pulpy paste. Smooth that on your face and lie down for a few minutes. You can also just slice the peaches and put them on your face. This is an instant pick-me-up for your skin because of the vitamin C in the peaches. If you do this for even a few minutes your skin will look fresh, soft, and plump."

● Want to get rid of your acne? Borrow some berries. "If you're not allergic to strawberries you can mash a few fresh ones with a spoon and add a spoonful of white yogurt. It might tingle, but don't be scared. Just wash it off after a few minutes and look fresh and gorgeous. If you do this once a week it can really control your breakouts."

● No one wants to have redness on her face. "I take an egg yolk and add a few drops of fresh lemon to it. Smear this on your face for a few minutes to get the red out."

● "If you want to tighten your face, use the egg whites with a drop of lemon in it. Before you shower smear this on your face down to your breasts."

● Cucumbers really do smooth and relax your skin. "My grandmother cut cucumbers and put them all over her skin and it worked. My mother uses this and looks like she's 50."

EMU 4 YOU

Over twenty-five years in film, TV, and print, makeup artist Robyn Weiss, who works for FOX TV in L.A., has done the faces of just about everyone in the business, including Constance Marie of *George Lopez*, Dorothy Lucey of *Good Day LA*, and *Scoop*, and our own Kym Douglas. Robyn gets up every day at 2:15 A.M. to be at the studio for the early morning show. She's a down-to-earth, no-nonsense artist who likes to use pure products, including emu oil, on her clients. Say what? Yes, emu oil.

Robyn explains, "A plastic surgeon who was on a show I was doing recommended it and I've been using it ever since." What exactly is it? Well, emu oil has long been used by the Aborigines of Australia to get rid of pain and swelling. More important, Robyn claims it has been proven to thicken skin. (Hollywood Beauty Speak: Thick skin equals younger-looking skin!) You can find emu oil at health-food stores and only need to put it on once a day before you go to sleep. Jenny McCarthy is also a fan. She tells us, "Emu is an oil that really penetrates the skin when most oils just don't do the job. This seeps right into your skin and removes the fine lines. It's cheap and awesome. I put it on like putting on deodorant."

BB Extra: Robyn Weiss has a few other great tips. "For tired, puffy eyes I sit with cold tea bags on my eyes for five minutes," she says. "For a gentle exfoliator, I mix sugar with my face cleanser. For a breakout, I hold tea tree oil on the pimple for a few minutes." Kym adds, "As I got into my 40s, I got pimples and wrinkles at the same time. That's when I started trying the tea tree oil dabbed on with a Q-tip. I held it on the blemish for a few minutes before going to bed. I swear that even the large, sore, cystic ones disappeared. The tea tree oil pulls out the bacteria and soothes the zit while healing the blemish, avoiding the flaking and scaling caused by so many teenage, over-the-counter products.

IMAGE MAKER:
OLGA LORENCIN-NORTHRUP

Yugoslavian-born skin expert Olga Lorencin-Northrup of Kinara Spa in West Hollywood, California, has transformed the faces of such Hollywood elite as Halle Berry, Naomi Watts, Annette Bening, Susan Sarandon, Jennifer Garner, Kate Hudson, and Katie Holmes, to name a few. In the first few seconds of meeting the warm and inviting Olga, we instantly saw what makes her such a hit with the women who want to look perfect! Olga's philosophy is simple: "Radiant beauty on the inside out." She practices what she preaches.

What is your favorite inexpensive or homemade beauty tip or product?

First, you need to find out if you have dry skin or oily skin. If you have oily skin, take two egg whites, a few drops of lemon, and one small drop of olive oil. Whisk together in a bowl, put on your face, and leave on for a few minutes. Rinse and your face will be tighter and your pores will be clean. For dry skin, mix up honey and yogurt. Put this on your face and then rinse.

What's a good beauty routine for your clients?

Exfoliating daily with lactic acids that are right for your skin and moisturizing with oil.

What is your secret antiaging tip?

Smaller portions, low carbs, and healthy eating are the best ways to prevent aging. However, this must be in balance with exercise because a restrictive diet that contains too much or too little food will definitely age you. Too much or too little exercise will age you as well! I'd also increase your olive oil or cod liver oil consumption. You will see your hair, nails, and skin shining and restored.

What sets a star, socialite, or true beauty—the girl that we all look at constantly—apart from the pack?

I can have 100 women come to me and say they want to have beautiful skin. I work with them, analyze and determine what kind of skin they have, and then tell them what they specifically need to do. A month later, 98 of the women will come back to me and say they look better, feel better, and have some improvement. The celebrity will come back and her skin is flawless. Why? She followed the instructions **exactly**. She will have religiously done everything in a regimented and determined way. Usually stars are very disciplined because they have to be—their paycheck and career depend upon it. The beauty that stands out among the others is always very informed, regimented and disciplined. It's not a secret formula; it's hard work.

What is your favorite health and diet tip?

My husband is a mountain climber. While doing some climbing he found some Goji berries that the tour guides in the mountains eat for energy and stamina. The berries are freeze-dried untouched by human hands and then sealed. They're high in antioxidants, control sugar levels, and have lots of amino acids. Plus, they're very easy to pack in your purse.

What is the biggest beauty blunder most women are guilty of committing?

They overmoisturize without exfoliating, which creates aging. You're not allowing the dead skin to fall off if you're not exfoliating correctly for your skin type. Think of a big, glass baking dish filled with leftover lasagna. It's late and you want to get the food off. So, you grab a rough sponge and scrub and brush. You tear all the food off the dish, rinse, and . . . and then take a closer look. You've left behind a few scratches on the glass. Or you could gently fill the glass baking dish with warm, hydrating water and let it soak for a while, letting food particles gently loosen so you can easily rinse later or the next morning. The latter is what the correct lactic acid does to your face. It gently exfoliates without tearing or causing redness.

What is one secret beauty or dermatology tip that you share only with your favorite clients?

There is no secret. If someone tells you that they have a secret, then RUN! It's about fine-tuning, being informed about your skin, and being diagnostic about your face.

GILMORE GLAMOUR

Just because she plays a "Gilmore Girl" named Rory doesn't mean twenty-four-year-old actress Alexis Bledel doesn't have some adult skin-care concerns. "You think this skin comes easy?" she asks, pointing to the ivory finish of her own face. Her tip is a skin-care lube job. "About once a week, I steam my face with pure olive oil," Alexis says.

"You just get a bowl of hot water, dab a little olive oil on your dry spots and let it do its work." (She cautions you to avoid breakout spots so you don't have pimple interruptus.) "It's an old trick that really works and your skin stays soft and line free," she says. And just in case grease is your word, foodie star Rachael Ray insists that her favorite product "EVOO," or extra virgin olive oil, can be taken out of the kitchen. "My mom puts EVOO in her hair, and even uses it to soften her feet!" Rachael tells us.

Alexis Vogel, who created gorgeous Pam Anderson's sexy kitten eyes, knows that you can't look your best if your peepers look tired and played. Her solution? "I take a potato and make thin slices. Put them right on your puffy eyelids and sit for ten minutes. It's an instant eye lift that I learned from a Polish beauty expert that I see," Vogel says. How does it work exactly? "My doctor says that it drains and pulls out the toxins from your lids while being very soothing and quite affordable at the same time." (By the way, Alexis found out that this treatment is kosher and can even help get rid of acne!) Please don't cry tears of joy now. You'll only get puffy.

SPOONING WITHOUT A MAN

Speaking of which . . . Want to reduce facial puffiness? Who doesn't? Just put a spoon in the freezer for a few minutes to reduce your punim—poof. Specifically, lay it over your eyelids and at the same time hold an ice cube against the roof of your mouth with your tongue. Please don't let anyone see you do this because they'll think you've lost your mind. They won't believe it when you tell them that the chill of the ice cube reduces the swelling in your face from the inside out.

FOOD FOR FACE—PART THREE

Okay, it's the night before Christmas. *Oops, sorry, wrong occasion.* It's the night before your big sashay-inducing shindig and you want to ensure that you will look your absolute best come morning. According to L.A.'s top naturopath/esthetician Karin U. Kanzler, eat these foods for immediate results: spinach, broccoli, and dark green veggies. (Okay, maybe pop a Gas-X first.) You want them because they're rich in minerals and vitamin A. In other words, these are your antidote to dry skin and wrinkles. Consume one serving daily of these super foods and you are bound to wake up looking like Charlize Theron, or at the very least the best version of you that you can be.

TEA FOR YOU

Here's a fast fix to percolate tired skin. If you have that dull, lifeless look to your epidermis, just brew a pot of chamomile tea, adding the juice of two lemons into the pot and two teaspoons of honey. Drink throughout the day. A-list celebs know chamomile calms the system and reduces inflammation brought on by stress and late nights on the Sunset Strip.

IMAGE MAKER: OCTAVIA ELLINGTON

At the Jim Wayne Salon in chichi Bev Hills, Octavia Ellington provides something better than Botox. Octavia's innovative concepts keep Hollywood's elite looking young and healthy. How? She prefers a holistic approach that pampers and replenishes the body, mind, and spirit. Her products are made from the highest quality aromatherapy and fruit-enzyme ingredients.

Clients who flash flawless faces include Mischa Barton, Katie Holmes, Nicollette Sheridan, Amanda Bynes, Kimberly Stewart, Elle MacPherson, Jennifer Capriati, Andy Roddick, Jennie Garth, Paula Abdul (hang on we're getting writer's cramp), Amber Valletta, Michelle Phillips, Rachel Hunter, Maria Shriver, and Laura Dern. To name a few.

What are your five favorite products in your bathroom right now?
Relaxing body wash, lavender essential oil, Frutta face cleanser, butt-firming cream, antiaging serum.

If you had only $100 to spend on products, what would you buy first?
Cleanser, daily scrub, day cream, and sunscreen.

What is the best antiaging tip you have?
First thing in the morning, drink an eight-ounce glass of organic vegetable juice. Also use Octavia Anti-Aging Serum.

Tell us about your biggest beauty blunder in life.
I was 15 years old. I put bleach in my hair and it all fell out!

Please tell us one secret beauty tip that you share only with your closest friends.
Octavia Super Face Peel. Left on overnight, it will have your skin glowing the next morning when you wake up. The vitamin A does wonders.

You Glow Gal

Another way to help you look great overnight is to drink fresh-squeezed vegetable juice with lemon juice and cayenne pepper. It will give you an instant rosy cheek effect. The vegetable juice boosts energy and the cayenne increases circulation for a healthy glow!

SOMETHING FISHY

She's been married and divorced more times (on TV!) than Jennifer Lopez, but it hasn't caused any fine lines on the gorgeous mug of Emmy winner Susan Lucci. La Lucci says that one of her biggest beauty secrets is sardines. Yes, sardines, so please let's say, "Go fish." Susan insists the fish oil helps her skin stay lubricated and moisturized. It will also make you glow from the inside out. Ask the experts, because it turns out that TV's Erica Kane is right on. According to a new study, large doses of vitamin D, found in sardines, halve the risk of developing colon, breast, and ovarian cancer. Professors at the University of California, San Diego, say that three to six servings of oily fish eggs, milk, and cod liver oil could save millions of lives. Author Jordan Rubin (*The Maker's Diet*) is also a big proponent of cod liver oil and touts its many health and beauty benefits.

Overheard on the Red Carpet: We've heard of weird divorce demands and fights to the death over the cat, the Rolls, and the Beverly Hills mansion. But what A-list couple, who dramatically hit the skids, tussled it out over their facialist? In the end, they worked it out with the appointment girl to make sure she never booked them on the same day. (*Now that we're not together, we can't both have our zits popped by the same hands on the same day!*) By the way, at $500 a session, she's no bargain—and we're talking about the facialist, not their divorce attorney.

WE'LL ALWAYS HAVE PARIS

There is no fooling around when you ask **Paris Hilton** for her beauty tips. First, she delicately wipes the cream cheese off her lips because she's devouring a gigantic bagel for breakfast on the Warner Brothers lot in Burbank. (The sight of all those carbs had Cindy and Kym passing out.) Second, she says words that in Hollywood might make the heavens part and the Hollywood Hills collapse. "I don't work out. I don't diet. I just have a good metabolism. I guess I'll start Pilates though—everyone does it." Digging deep inside,

Paris mulls over whether there are any actual tips she might have that real women can use. "Always wash your face before you go to bed. When people don't do that their skin gets really, really bad. So I always wash and then I use Crème de la Mer. It's really good stuff. It's hot." (Yes, we swear she actually said her catchphrase.) And with that she stuffed the rest of her bagel into her mouth, smiled, and teetered away on her three-inch platforms.

HOUSEWIFE HOTTIE

Felicity Huffman—aka Lynette on the megahit series *Desperate Housewives*—is the wife of acclaimed film actor William H. Macy and mom to a 3-year-old and a 5-year-old. It's no wonder, she laments, "I'm lucky if I have time to wash my face all day." Actually, Ms. Huffman has a little bit of time on her hands to use some great products on her porcelain skin. "I do a lot of moisturizing and I'm really into Leaf & Rusher," says Felicity. This new line was created by Norman Leaf, M.D., and Rand Rusher, R.N. It deals with the aging process of skin by using highly active forms of vitamins, algae, and messenger peptides to improve texture, tone, and clairty. (It's also good for the guys and won a recent award from *Men's Health* magazine.) Felicity insists, "I love their whole skin-care line, but I'm completely infatuated with this special face serum they carry. It just sucks into your skin. I look at my face after I put it on and it's almost like my skin is saying, 'Thank you, thank you, thank you.' " The product is called Active Serum, and it delivers Retinol combined with vitamin C. Felicity stopped there and actually asked *us* to reveal a tip. "What did Teri Hatcher say was her beauty tip?" (Hmmm, for that Felicity, you'll have to turn to page 156.) By the way, Leaf & Rusher also features a product we love called Green Tea Wash, a soap-free cleanser that quickly gets rid of makeup and impurities in the pores. It's made from licorice extract and green tea, and produces a natural glow that leaves us anything but desperate.

BB Extra: Lindsay Lohan and Marcia Cross swear by TX Lips by Leaf & Rusher.

QUEEN'S LOGIC

Queen Latifah doesn't mind making a royal proclamation: "I think if you wear makeup a lot of the time, it's really important to let your face rest as much as possible. Don't wear makeup at certain times of the day at all. Clean your face entirely and give your skin a break."

How does she get her flawless skin? "My grandmother turned me on to baking soda as an exfoliant. It's cheap and you just rub it around your face. It's very gentle and it works as well as any of the expensive products."

Finally, her royal subjects might like to know one more tip: "I hate soap. Throw away your soap," the Queen implores. "I've never used soap in my life. Dries your skin out, baby."

YO PLAY

Yogurt isn't just a better choice than a triple hot fudge sundae covered with wet walnuts. But we digress. Yogurt is also good for eliminating age spots and lightening what's known as a pregnancy mask. Why? Yogurt contains a natural bleach that helps lighten skin. Many top models regularly wash with plain white yogurt. Mix one teaspoon of yogurt with one teaspoon of pure honey. Rub on your face and then wash away.

SWEET STUFF

Young Hollywood hottie Jessica Biel (*Blade: Trinity* and *Stealth*) is a sweet girl from Colorado—and that's not just because of her sunny disposition and all those years she spent on *7th Heaven* as the character Mary. "I love to do sugar scrubs on my skin, but I never buy the expensive stuff they have in the department stores," Biel insists. "I just go buy a big bag of large-grain sugar. I put a teaspoon of it in my cleanser and then scrub away, but not too hard. It's a really cheap way to keep your skin looking clean and luminous." Biel admits that she's also a major moisturizer devotee. "I don't just moisturize my face and neck, but I go down into my cleavage. And I'm big on moisturizing my hands. . . . I'm actually seeing people drive around L.A. these days wearing little white gloves so their hands won't get tan while they drive. They're either saving their hands from aging or they're going to a very swanky tea party," she says, laughing.

BB Extra: Funny lady **Mo'Nique** has another unique skin-care tip. "I don't buy products with apple, orange, lemon, or melon extracts to put in my bath. I just take an apple, orange, lemon, or melon and cut slices. Then I throw them in my bath to smell great. They also soften my skin."

THEY'RE FEELING VERY SLEEPY

Okay, so it's not really the first time we've ever heard this, but it is coming from one of the greatest beauties ever from across the pond. According to **Catherine Zeta-Jones**, who is so pretty we want to scream, it's curling up with her pillow that gives her that happy, line-free look. "Sleep is the biggest beauty secret of all," she insists. The brunette beauty claims she and hubby **Michael Douglas** go to bed almost every night by 8:30 P.M. Being beauty mind readers, we know you're thinking, "Well, **Michael Douglas** is gorgeous, but he is over 50, so maybe he needs a little more sleep than the younger hunks . . . especially with **Catherine** a breath away." But **Lisa Rinna** and her *L.A. Law* hubby **Harry Hamlin** tell us that even on date night—aka Friday night—in La La Land, they go to bed no later than 9:30 P.M. We don't know if this means they immediately sleep-sleep or just sit up on their five-hundred-count sheets and talk, uh, world politics, but we don't ask those kind of questions.

Pimples, Punked

While testing twelve leading soaps (you know who you are) on acne bacteria, the Robert Wood Johnson Foundation in Princeton, New Jersey, found that the really expensive stuff didn't get rid of the zits. In fact, the most generic antibacterial liquid soap was proven the most effective pimple remedy. Remember that they said liquid. It seems that the antibacterial agents in the soap kill the creepy bacteria that cause the little eruptions in the first place.

SWEAT AND GLOW

Asian beauty and body beautiful **Michelle Yeoh** (*Crouching Tiger, Hidden Dragon* and *Memoirs of a Geisha*) says her beauty regimen is a two-step program—and her two tips don't cost much. "I believe in a lot of water. And I've been known to exercise more than once a day when I really want to drop a few pounds and make my skin glow at the same time. It really works. This way you're always spiking your metabolism, too."

OPRAH'S PHILOSOPHY

The **Big O** didn't pick raindrops on roses or whiskers on kittens as two of her favorite things. (Besides, she's a dog person.) On an episode of *The Oprah Winfrey Show* titled "Favorite Things," the most trusted name on TV said that she loves Philosophy's Hope in a Jar cream. (By the way, it's one of our favorites, too, as an economical and phenomenal beauty cream that makes fine lines disappear while making the need for foundation obsolete.)

JOY: TO THE WORLD

Actress-model Joy Bryant struts her stuff for The Gap and Victoria's Secret while starring in movies opposite Denzel Washington and 50 Cent. She certainly has the cash to buy expensive beauty products, but she prefers an all-in-one solution to just about everything. "I swear by Vaseline. It's the cheapest, most versatile product in history," Joy divulges. "If you have dry skin, smear it with Vaseline. If you want some shimmer on your eyes, put a layer of Vaseline instead of expensive eye shadow. I use it on my feet, my cuticles, and then I put some of the leftovers on a rag and shine my shoes with it. It's a huge, huge, huge part of my beauty regime." Joy admits that occasionally she will splurge on other products. "I love Dr. Brandt Microdermabrasion in a Jar. Ladies, it's the greatest thing since low-calorie sliced bread! It totally works. You can get it at Sephora. It's just the greatest exfoliant. You smear it on and boom, boom, boom. I also like Peter Thomas Roth Anti-Aging Cleansing Gel." She jokes, "I'm really 40, but these products keep me young." (By the way, she's really in her late 20s.)

SPEAKING OF ZITS

Just in case you don't feel like plunking down your credit card on products, we can also offer a far less expensive way to deal with those teeny pimple mountains that are trying to take up residence on your face. You should cover your zit with regular white toothpaste—not the gel type. The white stuff has an agent in it that will dry the pimple in a matter of hours.

WHEN LIFE GIVES YOU LEMONS, SMEAR THEM ON YOUR FACE

Young star Evan Rachel Wood (*Running with Scissors*, *Across the Universe*, TV's *Once and Again*) doesn't believe in sour grapes even though Hollywood is a tough place. She believes in lemons. She uses them on her flawless skin to keep it in the best condition. "If I have a pimple or something creepy like that erupting on my skin, I just buy a fresh lemon. Not the lemon juice. You need the real lemon," she says. "I just cut open the lemon, dunk my finger into the juice and then put my clean finger on the zit. It dries it up overnight—and it always works. Try it."

THE MOST DEPRESSING NEWS WE'VE EVER HEARD

Want to keep your skin looking young? You'll have to cut down on sweet cakes, candy, and cookies. The sugar in them attaches to collagen, resulting in stiff, inflexible skin that makes wrinkles deeper and more noticeable.

Now excuse us while we eat a final Cinnabon and then go jump off a building to end it all.

Pore it on

Size does matter—and it could even give you better skin.

Sarah Jessica Parker's facialist has a great tip for those of us who prefer at-home, do-it-yourself-for-peanuts spa treatments. Yana, who goes by only one name, says you should match your face scrub with your pore size.

In other words, if the grains in your scrubby stuff are too small, they won't penetrate your skin. If they're too large, you can actually hurt your skin or make it red.

So you need a grain that's just right.

BB Extra: Ling Chan, facialist to **Uma Thurman**, cautions that too much scrubbing and exfoliating can actually irritate your skin. She reminds us that cream-based products that contain rounded microbeads are gentler than their more gritty counterparts. And while she's on the topic, Ling advises limiting the use of glycolic acid and AHA (alpha hydroxy acids) products to twice a month because they're too harsh to use with any greater frequency.

BB Extra: Don't use those grains on your lips. Too harsh! But you can easily get rid of the dead skin on your kisser by using a soft washcloth with warm water. Wipe gently and follow with a liberal slather of lip balm.

IMAGE MAKER: VICKI COOPER

Vicki Cooper runs Faces by Vicki in Beverly Hills, and this premiere makeup artist has a client list that has included Annette Bening, Ali MacGraw, Geneviève Bujold, Ally Sheedy, Daryl Hannah, and Finola Hughes.

What are your five favorite products in your bathroom right now?

I love Ecologica Soapless Cleanser. I would die without it! I also use Ecologica Eye Protective Serum, Ecologica Regenerative Cream, Borlind LL Bi-Aktiv Day Cream. I love this for the décolletage! I also use Advance Vitamin C Serum.

If you had only $100 to spend on products, what would you buy first?

The first thing that I would purchase is a good soapless natural cleanser followed by an organic moisturizer and eye cream. I don't believe in astringents or toners since they do nothing for the skin. Keep the products simple. You don't need to spend a fortune to have beautiful skin.

What's the best antiaging tip you have to share with us?

Stay out of the sun! The best beauty secret was taught to me by my mother. At 87, she looks about 60 thanks to staying out of the sun. Another secret is to drink plenty of water. Moisturizing the skin needs to start from within.

Share one secret beauty tip that you give only to your closest friends.

A trick that I have taught some of my actress and model clients who feel a blemish erupting before a photo shoot is to intermittently apply an ice cube for thirty seconds on the blemish. This helps it from coming to a head. A trick that I used when I had a reaction to a mosquito repellent in Jackson Hole, Wyoming, without products available was to dab toothpaste on the blemishes while sleeping. The toothpaste really helps dry the blemishes.

If you had only ten minutes to get ready what would you do?

Hmmm, ten minutes a day to get ready sounds like my average morning! I wash my face with the Ecologica Soapless Cleanser followed by the eye cream and moisturizer, brush my teeth, run a brush through my hair, and apply a beautiful lip color. Voilà!

What is your favorite at-home, in-a-quick-pinch home remedy for beautiful skin?

There are times when my sweet husband surprises me with an important social event with little notice to prepare. I indulge by applying my protein-enzyme masque and peel to my face. This is the same treatment I prepare for my clients who attend the Academy Awards and need to look their best on the red carpet. Afterward, my face is smooth and glowing. Makeup simply glides on and I look and feel years younger.

DROPPING IT

Your limo has pulled up on the driveway to whisk you off to the People's Choice Awards or the local PTA meeting, and true disaster strikes. On your 200th glance in the mirror, you spot a zit that seems to have erupted in mere seconds. Short of major plastic surgery, what to do, what to do? First, gently place an ice cube on the problematic pimple for a few seconds and then immediately (but gingerly) press a cotton ball soaked in eye drops on the mini mountain. This works because the ice combined with the drops will make your blood vessels contract, alleviating the redness. A dab of cover-up later and you're ready for your close-up.

STEAM IT UP, BABY

Gorgeous actress Sanaa Lathan has starred in *Blade*, *The Best Man*, *Love & Basketball*, and *Disappearing Acts*. But when she wants to get her hot bod and beautiful face ready for love scenes with Wesley Snipes, Omar Epps, and Simon Baker, she does what she dubs her "sauna trick." "I go to a sauna once a week and do ten-minute intervals," Sanaa tells us. "I sit in the heat for only ten to fifteen minutes, tops, but you can adjust based on your own tolerance. Then I get out and take a cool to cold shower or jump in a cold pool. Next, I go sit in the sauna for another ten minutes followed by another cold shower or dip in the pool. I keep alternating for an entire hour."

The end result? "It's amazing for your skin," Sanaa insists. "It also gets rid of water weight and gives you the same endorphin rush you'd get from running."

"When you're all done, your entire body will be tingling, you'll feel entirely relaxed, and people who see you will say, 'Wow, your entire being is glowing. What did you do? Wow! What are you rubbing on your skin?'" she says with a laugh. "I just say, 'I run hot and cold.'"

Yes, They Were Fat and Didn't Go to Their Proms

Perhaps you're feeling a little bit unsure about your own beauty potential. Those who walk the red carpet on a regular basis have the same nagging doubts and fears. In a hushed voice, we asked the world's most beautiful to tell us what they don't like about themselves when they stare into that horribly unforgiving full-length mirror.

This might make you feel a little bit better:

Tyra Banks: "My eyebrows are too far apart. I'd love to have longer eyelashes and a wider smile like **Julia Roberts** or **Cameron Diaz**. My mouth is small and tight. My calves are nonexistent, so I rarely wear skirts or shorts. And I have cellulite, not just on my booty, but on my arms."

Eva Mendes: "I have this huge overbite. My siblings used to call me Bugs."

Michelle Pfeiffer. "Ever since I was a teenager, I thought that I had duck lips."

Ashlee Simpson: "I have a big nose, though I love it. I've got a hump on it and everything."

BB Secret: A short time later, according to recent tabloid photos, the hump is gone. In Hollywood, love is so fickle.

Feel better about yourself now?

CHAPTER 3

Why Can't We Air Kiss and Makeup?

Doesn't everybody just want one thing in life...longer eyelashes?

—**Eva Longoria**

Maybe you'll never make the Grammy Awards. Maybe you'll never make a movie or a magazine cover. But you can still star in your own life. The secret is to bring out your own natural beauty. Enhance, enhance, enhance! Because when you do, you bring out more than just good looks. You bring out your own natural confidence, too.

—Celebrity makeup artist **Alexis Vogel**

Nothing is as beautiful as confidence.

—**Katie Couric**

As if their multimillion-dollar salaries aren't annoying enough, A-list celebs also have the best makeup artists giving them good face—and the best possible tips for when the above-mentioned makeup artist is doing something totally annoying like spending time with her own family or sleeping. We decided celebs couldn't continue to hoard these life-changing, face-altering wunder-suggestions. We wanted to know which products were a tiny piece of heaven. What can make anyone with a blush brush and a little mascara look like she's ready for the runway of her own life? *The Black Book of Hollywood Beauty Secrets* goes where no beauty book has gone before by giving you the most fabulous, cutting-edge tips. Just trying a few of the following fabulous suggestions will make a huge difference. Now, if we could only give you a tip that would allow you to make $20 million a (digital) picture . . .

KISS MY 8×10 GLOSSIES

Finally, we can watch something that wiggles or jiggles in a good way and has nothing to do with cellulite. In other words your best lip color might be something in your kitchen. Jell-O. Yes, Jell-O can be used as a lip stain that will last all day long. This is a supermodel tip often used in exotic locales including *Sports Illustrated* swimsuit shoots. To do the Jell-O lips, just dip a Q-tip into water and then into strawberry Jell-O powder. Your pout will be pink and you can kiss your leading man with abandon without smearing him with lipstick. O-O-O indeed.

YOU REALLY HAVE ARRIVED

With all the Learjet travel she does on a weekly basis, Jessica Simpson should look a little more haggard. But there she is sweeping through LAX looking fresh as a Daisy Duke. How? Why? Does she have a makeup genie in her bag? No, but here's a trick that Jessica does herself in the airplane lavatory. "I swipe a nude pencil along my inner eyes to brighten my eyes before I get off the plane," she tells us. Poof! Instant wake-up to face the paparazzi!

THE BLUSH LIFT

Still applying color to the apples of your cheeks? Swear on the life of your publicist that you'll stop right now! If you apply the blush higher, starting about an inch under the middle of the eye and extending it out over the top of the apples, "it visually pulls everything up," making you look younger, says NYC makeup artist Sue Devitt, who has used the trick on Sheryl Crow. "It makes you look as if you've had a natural face-lift.

BB Extra: And if you want to feel the blush even in those drab months when you winter in Sun Valley next to Kurt and Goldie, you can come to your own blah skin's res-cure. If you use a cream or powder blush in pink or peach during winter months it will create a natural-looking and much healthier flush to your skin. This is what Claire Danes's makeup artist does for her during the cold New York months.

Master Your Mascara

Boys do make passes at girls with long lashes. Just ask **Eva Mendes**, who is known for her luxe ones. How can yours look just as great?

Rule one: There are times to pump yourself up, but putting on mascara is not one of them. Resist the temptation to pump the wand into the tube. You won't get more mascara on the wand, but you will drive air into the tube, drying out the mascara. Pull out the wand, look for clumps on the end and wipe them off with a tissue. Then line up the wand under your top lash line. Wiggle the wand back and forth as you pull it up through your lashes.

IMAGE MAKER: STEEVE DAVIAULT

Teri, Lindsay, Keira, and Kate. Oh my.

We found a wonderful jewel named Steeve with all those *e*'s and he does 'em all. He makes the mugs of Teri Hatcher, Keira Knightley, Kate Hudson, Tom Cruise, and Lindsay Lohan look even more heavenly.

What is your favorite inexpensive beauty tip or product?

RoC Retinol Actif Pur Day and Night. I've also discovered some of my favorite tools in the discontinued products baskets at the cash register. Worth checking out.

What are your all-time, never-fail, top-five best beauty products that you can't live without?

I love Visiora by Dior, which you can only find in specialty beauty stores. Highlighter from Kanebo, Mentha Lip Shine by C.O. Bigelow, Bad Gal Lash Mascara by Benefit, or for more natural lashes, Shu Uemura mascara, Revolution tinted body moisturizer by DuWop, Veil Foundation Primer by Bodyography, or Laura Mercier Foundation Primer.

You have only $100 to spend on products. What is on your list?

Laser in a Bottle by Dr. Brandt.

What is the most unusual item you've ever used on yourself or someone else?

Crushed raspberries for cheeks and chocolate for the lips.

What is the craziest thing you've ever done for beauty?

Botox! I love it.

Liner Notes

Celebrity makeup artist Lisa Williams-Fanjoy gives good face to Academy Award winners, sports celebrities, musicians, and many beautiful daytime actors and actresses like *The Young and the Restless* star **Eileen Davidson**. She says that the key for many of her stars is a lip color that lasts the entire day. "I use a lip liner pencil in a nice, natural shade. Line the lips. Then color the whole lip area with the same pencil. Add gloss or lipstick over the lined lips and your lips will look 'done' all day long."

BB Extra: Lisa also says that the natural glow her clients use to shine on set comes from a very inexpensive place. "In a pinch, just jump in a warm shower, towel dry, and then apply baby oil all over your skin. It gives you a dewy, luminous appearance."

OIL, BLACK GOLD, TEXAS TEA

Tom Pecheux, the French makeup artist who pretties the fabulous faces of **Nicole Kidman** and **Uma Thurman**, says not everything in his makeup kit is high-end. One of Pecheux's favorites is a $4 tube of Johnson's Baby Oil Gel. He tells us he uses it just about everywhere on his models and clients—on the lips, the hands, and the elbows. It's great for layering over eye shadow to set your look.

LOW BROW

Elisha Cuthbert, gorgeous as Jack Bauer's daughter on the hot show *24*, doesn't focus on a certain part of her anatomy 24-7. "If you go and get your eyebrows waxed, don't touch the top of them," warns **Elisha**. "That's where the shape sort of comes in. You have to speak up, because you don't want anyone to butcher your brows." **Elisha** got this good advice from her mother.

BB Extra: *Boston Legal* star **Lake Bell**, who has been linked to hunky bad boy **Colin Farrell**, insists that she never lets anyone touch her famous brows. "If you've got big brows like I do, you've just gotta own it. I don't wax mine."

HIGH BROWED

Damon Roberts does not pluck around. Ask him the most crucial part of a woman's (or a man's) face and he answers in approximately three seconds. "The eyebrows are the most important feature on the face. They're also the most underestimated part of your body. I call a good brow job the five-minute face-lift. If you can't do anything else, get your brows done," Damon tells *The Black Book*.

"Your brows bring structure to your face and make you look more alert," says Damon, who doesn't want to brow drop, so we'll just tell you that he has perfected the arches of Madonna, Mandy Moore, Vanessa Williams, Reba McEntire, and Molly Simms to name a few screen and stage beauties who will never be browbeaten.

So now that you know that your brows need help, what does Damon suggest? Get out your tweezers, brow scissors, and powder (or just order one of his Damon Roberts Eyebrow Kits) and follow along here.

● "My best advice is to go a little thicker with your brows," Damon says. "Thinner brows age everyone. Plus, the thinner brow makes you look harsh and stern. When your brow is a little fuller, it's softer and prettier." Even the fairy-tale babes knew this to be true. "Look at Snow White. She always had the fuller brows while the Wicked Witch had the thin brows. Cinderella had fuller brows while the Evil Stepmother had thin brows. If you thinned out Cinderella's brows, she would look a little evil and certainly much more tense—so avoid thin brows!" Damon implores.

● That said, the old Brooke Shields "I'm wearing a small vermin-like crittter above both eyes" look is dead. "Real thick like Brooke used to have will never come back," Damon says.

● He says that you shouldn't go to your brow job with a picture. "Don't copy the brows of a movie star. Go for the best shape for your personal features," he insists. "What works for Madonna or Mandy will not work for everyone else. Just go in to a good brow artist and let them sculpt. Don't go in with a picture saying, 'It has to be this.'" He says good brows are like a black cashmere sweater. "Once you find the right style, the sweater and the brows will never go out of style. They will never be the wrong shape because both are timeless."

● By the way, he says that you should visit your brow specialist monthly. "You can clean up stray hairs in between appointments, but leave the basic shape to a professional."

● He cautions that if you don't have to do it . . . don't do your brows at home. "If you must do them at home, remember that less plucking is more."

● He says that those with transparent or sparse brows should color them in. "If you use a pencil, it has to be soft and subtle. I'm actually more in favor of powder on the brows. It's more natural looking, wears better, and if you're perspiring, then it settles in more." He adds, "A pencil looks harsh. If you go too dark, it looks terrible."

- And if you dye your hair (as if anyone doesn't) then should you also color your brows? Damon suggests, "If you're blonde, go two shades deeper for your brows. If your blonde brows are too light they will wash you out, and you need some color to frame your face. If your hair is really dark, go one or two shades lighter to lighten up your face."

- And finally, he says that once you get a brow job, you will never go back to a wild jungle over your eyes or look like two gremlins are sitting on your face.

Low Brow

We all know about the hair-enhancing formula for balding men called Rogaine. But here's a little insider tip for the ladies from a top celebrity makeup artist who tells us that many of his female and male stars use Rogaine on their eyebrows to add fullness and shape the natural way. This is especially helpful if you're a little light in browland or got a little tweezer crazy. It's not an overnight treatment, but takes about six months for full bloom. And in the interest of not hurting yourself on the road to beauty, please be careful and not get any drops of Rogaine into your eyes.

IMAGE MAKER: CAROL SHAW

Kym sat down with Carol Shaw at the swanky, beachfront Shutters Hotel in Santa Monica, California. As they enjoyed organic, prewashed berries and two cups of herbal, unsweet-ened tea, the long, lean, blonde Carol spilled some organic makeup secrets.

By the way, Carol is the founder of Lorac Cosmetics and has a clientele of A-list women in her chair that would make anyone's head swivel. She gets cheeky with Nicole Kidman, Debra Messing, Susan Sarandon, Geena Davis, Naomi Campbell, and Lucy Liu to name a few luscious luminaries.

What are a few beauty secrets you share only with your closest friends?

Get coconut oil in solid form and let it soften to normal temperatures. Then put it in your hair. Also, I use tweez-ers to pull off pieces of dead skin on my face after micro-dermobrasian.

What has been your biggest beauty blunder?

I suffered from severe cystic acne and had reddish skin problems all over my face when I was a teenager. I'd go out and buy this thick, chalky paste-like foundation a friend told me to buy. It had a lot of red color in it and I'd put it on like a mask. When I went out of the house I looked like a woman covered in a mask of Pepto-Bismol! Yuck!

What is the biggest beauty mistake you see most women make again and again?

Women either don't use enough makeup or they use too much makeup. It's the same problem. Remember that a lit-tle color goes a long way. It takes very little makeup to look beautiful. Then I'll see these women walking around and I think, "Would it kill you to put on a little lip gloss and some concealer?"

Feeling Blue?

"Ain't no hollaback girl" **Gwen Stefani** has that megawatt smile thanks to a layer of sheer light-blue gloss that she wears over that va-va-voom lipstick. The coolness of the blue brings out the whiteness of her teeth.

SHE LOVES IT . . . AND SO DOES SHE

Jennifer Love Hewitt has been a star since childhood and could afford any gloss her lips desired. Yet, her Bonne lies over her smacker. "My Bonne Bell lip gloss is about seventy-five cents and I have worn it to almost every main Hollywood event for the past two years," she says. Talk about lip service. Before she goes live with Reege, Kelly Ripa needs a little morning, post-feed-the-kiddies pick-me-up that screams, "I am one sexy mama." What does the trick? Ripa says, "I like to put on a sheer-red gloss like Too Faced Fat Kiss in Fat Jelly. It brightens your face and makes your teeth look whiter."

BB Extra: By the way, Too Faced also makes an extraordinary lip plumper. Too Faced Lip Injection super-sizes your kisser as much as 20 percent by really stimulating blood flow to your lip area. (See chapter 5 for more uses of this product!)

Multiplaction Tables

You've heard the Tinsletown adage "Everyone uses everyone." Well, when it comes to beauty supplies, we amend that to "Everything can be used for everything." Let us explain: You can use your foundation for your face, but it's also a perfect lip primer and eye shadow base, and if you have some dark spots on your body, then a dab will do you on your gams or arms. You can also wash off your old mascara wand, put some of your light beige foundation onto it, and comb the foundation through the hairline around the face. An inexpensive touch-up for your hair. We're all really natural blondes anyway, right?

BRIGHTY WHITIES

Let's say you're on your way to Spago and glance in the BMW mirror only to gasp in horror. No, it's not **Anna Nicole Smith** and a new male senior citizen in the car behind you. It's that your teeth are an unsightly yellowish color indicating too much Starbucks or unfamiliarity with a dentist. The solution: Use food-grade hydrogen peroxide. *Poseidon* star **Emmy Rossum** does. "It tastes terrible," she tells Cindy. "But it really does the job." Celebs use it before going in front of the camera. They run it across their teeth and then do a quick swish around the mouth before spitting. Do not swallow. Do this after drinking your soy, no-fat, vanilla latte or after downing a glass of red wine, and your teeth will suddenly look shiny white again. Remember, do not swallow. It's a cheap way to get a bright smile without spending $1,000 at the dentist.

Overheard on the Red Carpet: What sexy hunk of the moment is so obsessive about his pearly whites that brushing has become his mistress? He scrubs his teeth no less than ten times a day. Girlfriends claim they find toothbrushes—manual and electric—all over his house. He even keeps one in the glove compartment of his luxury car.

LASHING OUT

Your publicist is having a snit because you're in the latest edition of *Us* on the arm of one of those *Entourage* boys. Your agent hasn't returned your calls in days. Just when you can't take any more pressure, you notice that your eyelashes aren't curvy, upswept, and beautiful, but flat, straight, and looking like you just completed a few days of community service for . . . well, we don't want to talk about that. To combat flat lash, put some hair gel on a pipe cleaner mascara wand. A little goes a long way. Now, curl your lashes and then coat them with the gel. Let the gel dry and then put on your mascara. The gel will not only hold the mascara, but will also keep your lashes pointing toward the heavens.

IMAGE MAKERS: LAURA DELUISA AND CRISTINA BARTOLUCCI, COFOUNDERS OF DUWOP COSMETICS

Together they've created perfect faces for Bruce Willis, Ben Stiller, Tim Robbins, Keanu Reeves, and Jennifer Garner. How did two girls get so lucky? Well, it sounds like a Hollywood movie: years ago, Laura and Cristina ran into each other on the set of an NBC show and started the DuWop line in Laura's kitchen. Today it's one of the hottest among celebs.

What are your five favorite products in your bathroom right now?

Cristina: Matty's Skincare Skin Prep Cleanser, DuWop's Reverse Eyeliner, Philosophy Booster Shots, DuWop's Lash Lacquer, and a Shu Uemura eyelash curler.

Laura: Matty's Skincare Purely C Vitamin C Serum and Energizing Skin Complex, ARTec Color Depositing Shampoo, DuWop's Hands2Hair, and DuWop's Blush Therapy in Retreat.

If you had only $100 to spend on products, what would you buy?

Cristina: Maybelline's Great Lash Mascara, a neutral pink lipstick that can be used on lips and cheeks, an amber/gold eye shadow, a cherry ChapStick, a day/night cream, pHisoderm cleanser, and an eyelash curler.

Laura: My skin-care products. I would buy a cleanser, moisturizer, toner, and Vitamin C Serum from Matty's

Skincare. It's all well priced and the most important part of my beauty regime.

Give us your best antiaging tip.
Cristina: Intensive eye cream.
Laura: Eight hours of sleep and drinking lots of water.

What is one secret beauty tip you share only with your closest friends?
Cristina: After you have applied your makeup, dip your blush brush into your blush, then sweep it over your eyes. This will make them pop.

If you had only ten mintues to get ready, what would you do?
Cristina: Blend a tinted moisturizer all over my face and neck, apply two coats of black mascara, dab a light pink blush on the apples of my cheeks, and finish it off with a neutral-colored lip gloss.
Laura: I usually only take ten minutes to get ready. I wash my face, apply moisturizer, mascara, and then Butter-cream Lip Balm.

What's your favorite in-a-quick-pinch, at-home beauty remedy?
Cristina: Plain white sugar is the most amazing body ex-foliator. I keep a jar of white sugar next to my bathtub and it leaves my skin glowing.
Laura: I use a natural-cloth scrub to exfoliate my body and buff away dead skin.

What's the biggest makeup blunder most women make and how can they fix it?

Cristina: I don't like it when women don't blend their foundation/tinted moisturizer/bronzer over their jawline and down their neck. It looks really unnatural. We created Revolotion, a tinted body moisturizer, so you can have the same skin tones on your complexion and body. You would apply your tinted moisturizer for the face all over your face and neck, and then apply Revolotion for the body from the neck down.

Laura: I don't like to see women with dark lip liner and pale lip color inside. We created Neutral Lip Pencils for this reason, as we believe your lip pencil should be neutral in color and be used to fill in your lips and act as a base for your lip color.

SHE GIVES GOOD FACE

Stand-up comic Monique Marvez, who has a hot new sitcom called *Shore Things* and a bestselling book called *Not Skinny, Not Blonde*, had her lean years while doing stand-up across the country. "I'm one of those lucky people who has acne and sensitive skin at the same time," she tells us. Yet, she found a great makeup trick that really works. "For years, I used Johnson's Baby Powder as my translucent powder. I'd put it over my foundation and it would absorb, but it never turned dark. Plus, it didn't have an offensive scent." Monique says that the savings were incredible. "I loved the baby powder. If it's good enough for a baby's ass, it's good enough for my face."

BB Extra: Just in case you're allergic to the talc, Burt's Bees has a talc-free powder that we love.

IT'S SICLICAL

Olé, Hispanic beauties. We did a tiny interview with Rea Ann Silva, a Beverly Hills makeup artist who regularly works on the faces of Alicia Silverstone, Kerry Washington, Jennifer Garner, and Sarah Michelle Gellar to name a few. She told us a great tip about how models sit around at shoots all day sucking on cherry popsicles because they're only ten calories and they stain the tongue in a gorgeous way. The popsicles also stain your lips a pretty natural pink and freeze the interior of your mouth, which helps to reduce any puffiness or swelling in the face from the inside out.

Liner Notes

It's not like we want you to toss out your black or brown liner, but it's time for an eye opener. Buy a dark gray or cobalt blue eyeliner (Chanel makes a great one) and give yourself a few fine lines around your eyes. These colors are guaranteed to stand out and make your eyes the main focus of your face like they do for Sienna or Angelina.

FROM DOWDY TO DIVA—PART ONE

Jeanine Canter, top Beverly Hills makeup artist to stars including Sela Ward and Maria Shriver and socialites including Ivana Trump, does a beauty speed round with us . . .

Tip-a-palooza: "The fastest and cheapest way possible to look great is to buy false eyelashes, trim them so they're custom fit to look just a little longer than your own lashes, and adhere. You will look glam in two seconds."

Cheapest product she loves: Maybelline eyebrow pencils. "The consistency can't be beat and they will never ever turn your brows orange."

Skip: Don't waste your cash on designer brushes that often cost $30 a pop. "My favorite tools are cotton balls and Q-tips. They're fresh each time and you can just throw them in the garbage when you're done."

Do it: "Before you put your eyeliner on, if using a brush or Q-tip, dip it into water then put the liner on. Water gives you staying power with any of your makeup."

Favorite product to save your skin: "To remove makeup, I always use Almay pads. Everything comes off in one swipe."

THE AA LIST

Up-and-coming actress Amy Adams—nominated for an Oscar for *Junebug*, and star of Will Farrell's campy comedy *Talladega Nights*—likes to give 'em lip service but refuses to spend too many pennies on having the perfect pucker. "One of my favorite cheap beauty tricks is Dr Pepper Lip Smackers, which cost about $1.29 at Target. I give a bunch of these every year for Christmas and all of my friends love them. They taste like Dr Pepper and the best part is that it gives you the perfect natural-looking gloss." Bonne Bell also has a great cheap gloss. Try it, try it, try it.

Overheard on the Red Carpet: Here's a fun little superstitious tidbit. A Brazilian Hollywood beauty who has become very wealthy, very fast in Tinseltown secretly confides to friends that one of the reasons for her financial success has nothing to do with her sexual prowess with wealthy studio heads or her unwavering and constant self-promotion. It really stems from her belief in old Brazilian folklore that she will never bag. Specifically, never ever ever put your purse (Hollywood Speak: IT BAG) on the floor in a restaurant. It will make you poor. That will make you frown. And then you will be poor and have wrinkles. We're going to sit down and grab a cold compress right now.

BB 911: **Erika Christensen**, star of *Flight Plan* and *Traffic*, says that she has taken a beauty misstep or two in her life. "Two words: brown lipstick," she says. "I guess there is a way to do it right, but it's not easy. I remember when I was 14, I would wear brown lipstick and I looked like I had smeared dirt all over my lips." **Erika**'s best tip these days: "Get a tan. I'm known as the Pale One. So, I try to get a little bit of color by going outside in the sun for just a few minutes. Also, I'm not always going to have time to do a major makeup job. So the solution is just a little bit of lip gloss and a great pair of sunglasses."

SHEER GENIUS

It's not that we're saying a nude Kate Hudson is boring. But her naked lips are another matter.

Paul Starr, makeup artist extraordinaire, says there's a trick he loves to use on the gorgeous actress. It seems that Kate is a huge fan of nude lips, but that can get a bit boring. Paul makes nude a little bit more racy by adding a little gold speckle to create texture on her lips or by rubbing some shimmery cream eye shadow on her kisser and topping it off with some gloss. It's a good way to jump-start your sexy smacker.

BLUSHING BEAUTY

If you're on the red carpet with a teeny tiny evening bag, it's hard to pack your entire makeup kit. Stars like Cameron Diaz know that you don't need to even try to cram your big blusher into your fabulous little Fendi. Just bring your favorite lipstick (not too dark) to double as a blusher.

BLACK BOOK TEEN SECRET!

She's, like, a junior league pretty woman. Emma Roberts—16-year-old gorgeous niece to superstar Julia Roberts—is playing Nancy Drew in a new film franchise about the girl detective. We decided to sleuth around ourselves to find out if Emma has any special beauty routines. "Are you kidding me!" she yelled into her cell. "I live for beauty!" Specifically, Emma says that she's already tending to her skin. "I really do care about moisturizing. It really is important at any age and my aunt Julia told me you're never too young to start putting on moisturizer. I use Dermalogica." She adds, "My face is so dry and tight that it hurts. The moisturizer really helps." Emma also told us that she's a little sick of how girls at her school "glop on too much makeup. Some girls wear so much base and bronzer that it looks like you could peel it off their faces. Ick." Her trick for staying natural looking? "Basically, I put on a little mascara, lip balm, and blush. Maybe if I'm going out I'll put on a lightly tinted moisturizer." And whose look would she like to try for just one day? "It's a tie between Rachel McAdams and Kirsten Dunst. They're so cute, plus they do good movies. I love them both so much." Emma also loves her little sister—even though the youngest Roberts has one request. "My little sister is always in my makeup bag. When I catch her, she will always say, 'But can't you just do a quick makeover on me!'" Emma admits that she has asked the same of someone who is pretty famous. "Aunt Julia has done makeovers on me and she's the best. She never puts on too much."

IMAGE MAKER: JESSICA LINDY, FOUNDER OF LALICIOUS

When her best glass jar of body scrub broke in the shower and ran down the drain, Jessica Lindy didn't cry. She just got some more jars and some cool ingredients and made her own new scrubs, like steamy Coffee Soufflé Body Scrub.

(Wakes you up; no caffeine!) When Jessica gave her one-of-a-kind mixtures to family and friends, they told her she should start her own line of products. Body Butters and Sugar Soufflé Scrubs were concocted in Jessica's kitchen with unique smells and tantalizing textures. Stars swear by the products like Coconut Cream Sugar Soufflé. Or maybe we should try the Passion Fruit Lime. Decisions, decisions.

What are your five favorite products in your bathroom right now?
LaLicious Brown Sugar Soufflé Scrub
LaLicious Vanilla Body Oil
Somme Institute face products
Comptoir Sud Pacifique Vanille Banane perfume
Too Faced Sun Bunny Bronzing Powder

If you had only $100 to spend on products what would you buy first?
Karite Lips Shea Butter Vanilla Lip Balm. I'm a lip balm fanatic. Klorane Dry Shampoo, I buy this stuff by the half case. It's the best dry shampoo out there!

What is your best antiaging tip?
Red wine, a positive attitude, a daily vitamin.

What's one secret beauty tip that you share only with your closest friends?
I'm having a tough time with this one because I share all my tips with everyone. But my best tip is to use bronzer. Whether you're fair or tan, bronzer always makes you look a little more alive.

What is your favorite in-a-quick-pinch, at-home beauty remedy?

Egg-white mask for your face. It tightens your pores in a snap!

Overheard on the Red Carpet: Yes, this is about hand jobs. What Hollywood star is so big that she just doesn't have time for a top Beverly Hills spa's regular overpriced massage? This ravishing redhead single-handedly invented and insisted on the Double Your Pleasure Four-Hand Massage. High-end salons and spas all over town heard the need and immediately complied. Now places like the trendy Sunset Tower Hotel in West Hollywood have on their spa services menu the Massage Four-Hands ($250) and the Hot-Stone Four-Hands ($375). Boon to her image for starting the trend . . . priceless!

CHAPTER 4

The Higher the Hair, the Closer to God

Sometimes my hair is a mess, and I can't find the right outfit and I feel like I weigh 300 pounds.
—**Cindy Crawford**, whom we think is just joking

My hair! He touched my hair.
—**John Travolta** to his head-bashing father in the classic film
Saturday Night Fever

The flat head is dead, and if you ask us, it's not a minute too soon. Unless you're 17, **Gwyneth Paltrow**, or you weigh ninety-eight pounds, it never really did do anything for anyone . . . so we say proudly, "The higher the hair, the closer to God" and finally Hollywood is agreeing. Fluffy, sexy, full hair is in—and please don't muck it up by snuggling up with your straight iron. Here are some of the best hair-care tips from the best tressed. Let's get it out of the way right here. **Jennifer Aniston** gets monthly trims, not cuts, but little trims. One tip down, a zillion to go.

Hey, Fatty

Yes, it's the e-mail you thought would never arrive: A producer spotted you at Target, took one look at you choosing which Q-tips are best, and now wants you to audition in six weeks for a plum role on *The OC*. Oh no! What will you do about your hair?

Consider this the truth hair bomb: Your locks depend on your lips. Yes, what you put into your stomach has a lot to do with the health of your mane. So start working from the inside out.

One important nutrient for healthy hair is gamma linoleic acid (GLA), which is an omega-6 fatty acid that fortifies your hair. Experts say that it's nearly impossible to eat enough of this acid through a regular diet, but you can buy supplements at nutrition stores. In six weeks your hair will be thicker and have more luster, promises Andrew Weil, M.D., author of *Healthy Aging*, who also knows the power of GLA.

Applying coconut oil directly to your hair also feeds your locks. The *Journal of Cosmetic Science* found that this yummy stuff helps fight protein damage to your hair. Researchers have discovered that this particular tropical oil is one of the few that actually penetrates the hair shaft and bonds to the protein. And you need to use it only once weekly for a thirty-minute session before shampooing. We recommend using only it on the ends of your hair because it can make your scalp a little too flat and oily.

Overheard on the Red Carpet: What hair goddess—whose naturally lush locks are coveted by everyone—is telling friends that her natural hair is not so natural and is the result of sewn-in extensions? After a short period, she found the fake hair was killing her own real hair. Now she tells everyone to go with what you were given and grow it out yourself.

IN A TIZZ OVER FRIZZ

Your agent has just called (or your girlfriend or coworker) and you're on the run to a chic lunch spot like Newsroom Café on Robertson. But your troublesome hair is not cooperating and frizz is setting in to ruin your entrance. Colorist Marie Robinson of the Sally Hershberger Downtown Salon in NYC says that the solution is in your purse, not your medicine cabinet. Marie recommends taking out your ChapStick—yes you read this right—dabbing it on your fingers, then running it through your hair to tame the flyaways and the frizz. It's a great tool when you're running around for the day because you can slip it into the teeniest Tod's bag. And frankly, after buying the Tod's, it helps to save some money on cheap tress smoothers.

Don't Let It Snow

Feeling flaky? Here's a quick tip. Crush up an aspirin and mix it with your regular shampoo. The properties in the aspirin will get rid of the dryness in your scalp, and suddenly your own personal snowstorm warnings will be history.

We should also mention that aloe vera gel not only works as hair gel with medium hold but gently moisturizes your scalp, without making it oily, to prevent dandruff.

BB Extra: Rub a dollop of aloe vera gel onto your legs before shaving. You'll avoid razor burn and your legs will feel silky and smooth.

Overheard on the Red Carpet: What A-list celeb has no horse sense? Trying on Alexander McQueen pony skin pumps in NYC, she called over the store manager to make sure no ponies were harmed in the making of her pumps. He had to assure this little blonde Oscar nominee that National Velvet, Seabiscuit, and even My Little Pony's heirs weren't hurt.

IMAGE MAKER: JONATHAN ANTIN

"Oh my God, it's just another calm day in my life," says superstylist to the stars Jonthan Antin. Frankly, his schedule is making us want to clutch our hair, although we never would because he would probably be very upset. Jonathan says, "I just finished a head. On camera. I'm talking to my manager. Doing a photo shoot. A client just walked in. And I'm talking to you at the same time." (Thank you, Jonathan, because we love your show *Blow Out!*)

Then there's the shrill ring of his cell phone. It's not an emergency from Madonna, Kirsten Dunst, Alicia Silverstone, Kate Bosworth, Ricky Martin, or Tiger Woods—just a few of his bold-faced clients. It's a honcho from Victoria's Secret wanting him to try out their new shampoo. "Did I smell it? Yes," Jonathon says into the phone. "I used it four times. I can't say anything else. I need to use a product seventy times before I'm sure." (His own product line, including the popular Dirt, sells out all over the country and his show *Blow Out!* is a hit in forty-five countries. The guy is so darn busy that he needs to spend two days reading his e-mails. "Some are so inspiring they make me cry like a baby," he says.)

Of course, *The Black Book* wouldn't let the conversation with the amazing Jonathan go flat, and he told us these tips:

- ***Don't be afraid to change your look.*** "Women have this element of, 'If it works don't fix it' when it comes to their hair. But I say go for a change. Hair should be fun. It's the only thing on our bodies we can change quickly, and it will come back. So, risk it. Remember that life is short and you can't be afraid to try new things."

- ***You can fight frizz.*** (Of course, this was a totally self-serving question because Cindy lives in Chicago, where her hair is in constant revolt.) "In Chicago, Atlanta, Houston, and Tampa, you have that humidity, which is bad for hair. What you do depends on what kind of hair you have. If you have straight hair you're fine. Just throw in a great volumizer and go out into the humidity. If you have fine hair that tends to frizz then let's start from the beginning because frizz doesn't start in the mirror with a blow dryer. It starts in the shower. Don't use a crummy or damaging shampoo that's full of detergent. Mine are sulfate free. You need a shampoo with pure essential water in it."

● *Wash with clean water, including a new filtration system.* "It's bad news, but if you're in the shower for an hour, that's the equivalent of pouring a gallon of chlorine on yourself and your hair," he says. "If you purify your water you don't have to worry. It's like bathing in a mountain spring."

● *And if you can't afford a purification system then just buy a few bottles of Evian or Fiji water, among other bottled products.* "For twenty years, I've been telling celebs to use bottled water to wash their hair before a shoot or a big event. It makes a huge difference," he says. "You can use a bottle of $2 pure water, too, before you go to a big event. It really makes your hair beautiful."

● *And finally, who has the best hair in Hollywood?* Jonathan laughs and says, "Well, Naomi Watts has amazing hair. Kate Bosworth is a national treasure of hair. But Madonna? She's queen of the hair world! I'd take my scissors and brush to her any day."

*And what celeb would he like to sit in his chair? "Donald Trump! Call me, Donald!" Jonathan says with a laugh.

SEX AND THE NITTY GRITTY

We'd love to hate **Kristen Davis** because she's beautiful, but frankly who has time? We're too busy watching her on reruns of *Sex and the City*. (We're still so glad she married Harry and kept all of Elizabeth Taylor's puppies. If you have to ask, it's not worth explaining.) We still asked: What's up with your hair and how do we get it? (Kym actually met her years ago in an acting class and says **Kristen** is a natural beauty, super focused, and has brass.) "First of all, I drink a lot of water, which keeps your hair beautiful. That's super important," **Kristen**, our NBF (Hollywood Beauty Speak: New Best Friend—known her for years, but have never spoken to her), insists. "And then I wash with Kérastase because my hair is beaten up so badly on sets and it's really gentle and moisturizing." She also has a secret trick for lovely locks. "I buy palm nut oil from South America [you can find it at health-food stores]. It was actually discovered by the tribes in the Amazon and the oil helps these people sustain a good diet. What I've found is it's magical as even a daily hair conditioner. It doesn't weigh your hair down and it makes it super shiny. Any girl with long hair needs to try it."

BB Extra: By the way, **Kristen**, Ronald Braso, a top stylist for genius Frederic Fekkai, also says that wheat germ oil is a fantastic summer conditioner. He begs his beach- or winter cruise–going clients to buy wheat germ soft gels. To use them on your hair, you simply break the gel apart, rub the oil into your hands and then smooth it on your hair. Look for the cold-pressed wheat germ oil that the best tressed have used for years.

Overheard on the Red Carpet: What high-powered hair guru gets between $3,000 and $6,000 to go to his celeb clients' houses or hotel rooms for "services rendered." He even giggles to himself that A-listers pay his $6,000 house-call fee. He brags that he walks in, takes one look at the nervous starlet, and tells her, "You're gorgeous. Just the way you are." Then he turns around on his Gucci moccasins and leaves, check in hand.

Letting It All Sink In

Deep condition your hair with product in the shower, then comb it through your locks. Why? In warm water, your hair will swell and absorb all of the ingredients. You want to make sure that you distribute the conditioner equally on your strands from top to bottom for maximum effect. Relax while the product sinks in fully and your hair absorbs all of its nourishing ingredients. Oh, and don't forget to wash out the comb. Dried product gets a little gunky.

A LOCK ON YOUR LOCKS

Love isn't the only thing that fades in a heartbreaking way if it's not treated right. When you leave the salon after getting a color treatment, your reds are on fire, and your blondes are as bright as the sun. A few weeks later, however, and it's like this Technicolor dream has done a slow fade and by the end of the month your hair color is dull and lifeless. Sob, sob, hair shouldn't be treated that way when all it does is give and give! The solution? A top Beverly Hills colorist tells us that heat is the biggest enemy to your color. She has her clients wash their locks with cool (not cold, we know you'll be howling) water and then blow-dry on a warm or even a cool setting. Try it for one month and you'll see your color go the distance.

HAIR APPARENT!

The pain is almost too much to bear. Why does fabulous redhead Julianne Moore always have super straight hair even when she's in the middle of a rainstorm on the streets of New York? (Quick story. Cindy once forgot to lock her bathroom stall at a press junket at the Essex House Hotel in NYC and JM walked in on her. "Oh my God!" screamed JM, "I'm so sorry!" . . . "Oh my God!" said Cindy. But instead of being truly horrified with her BCBG tights around her ankles, Cindy could only think, "Wow! That hair is just as good up close! And next time, I better lock the door unless perhaps George Clooney wants to walk in.") But we digress. JM's hair is enough to make most of us want to sit with our ball of frizzy hair on the kitchen floor, eat Oreos, and weep. But our little Miss Jules revealed one of her best hair secrets to us. "First of all, it's very easy to keep your hair straighter if you let it grow longer. I have a lot of hair and when it's shorter, it gets big and frizzy." (Thank God, she has actual hair problems!) "Actually, after I wash it, I just tie it back when it's wet into a ponytail. It pulls it tight and it just dries straight on me."

FROM THE HISTORY BOOKS

Did you know that in the year 1905 the average life expectancy in the United States was 47 years and that most women washed their hair only once a month, using borax or egg yolks for shampoo?! No wonder so many people lived far away in their own little houses way, way out on the prairie.

CATCHING UP WITH YOUR WAVES

There are many reasons why celebrities insulate themselves in their multimillion-dollar mansions all day long. The one that makes the most sense to us has to do with preventing the wind (or any other heinous element like the color-fading sun or, God forbid, the early morning mist called June gloom in Los Angeles) from ruining their hair.

The rest of us—we have to leave the house to earn a living. Yet why is it in your bathroom in the wee hours that your hair does those perfect cascading waves? But by the time the noon hour strikes, your waves might be flatter and more limp than . . . **Ricky Martin**'s career. The solution is to pack a mineral water spritzer in your bag. Sneak into a nearby bathroom when your locks look sad, mist up your waves, and rescrunch them by hand. The water will actually break the waves or the hydrogen bonds that you created in the morning and your hands can stage a hair do-over. By the time your locks dry again, you'll be doing a perfect afternoon wave.

SHINE IT ON

Want a simple trick to add shine to your hair? Run a silk scarf over your hair from the top of your roots to the (hopefully not split) ends. The scarf is full of positive charges that will jump onto your hair and make it shine.

BB Extra: Another shine trick is to add baking soda to your shampoo-lathered hair. The baking soda gets rid of old product glop, and once the residue is gone your natural shine will return.

(Tooth) Brush with Fame

Top New York stylists, instead of backcombing clients' hair to give it some lift, use a firm bristled toothbrush, digging it into the roots and teasing lightly. This quickly creates amazing volume. When you're done you can just spray with a light holding hair spray . . . or spritz the toothbrush with the hairspray before you tease. It cuts down on one of the steps, but don't go nuts with the hairspray or you'll turn your tease into a tangled, gunky mess.

WE DON'T WANT TO MISCHA HER

Okay, here's the skinny (literally) from the bathroom of **Mischa Barton** who has the loveliest long locks in the business. On the set of *The OC*, her hair gurus use a leave-in conditioner on her luscious mane and then towel dry her hair. Then they flip her hair over, blow-dry until it's only slightly damp, then roll her up in Velcro rollers for the set. The stylist will blow-dry again with a defuser—ten minutes on hot, ten minutes on cool. Finally, finally (we promise), the stylist simply removes the rollers and adds a drop or two of shine spray. Don't brush. Just run your fingers through your hair to get those perfect loose waves.

AND WHILE WE'RE ON THE GLAMAZON BABE TRICKS . . .

In New York City, salon king Ted Gibson helps to beef up Angelina Jolie's hair and turn it total sex kitten, with baby powder. Here's how you do it: After the initial prep with a shampoo, conditioner, and volumizer, set the hair with Velcro rollers and leave them in for fifteen minutes before removing. Then flip the head over and sprinkle a bit of baby powder into your follicles. Work a bit of it from your scalp all the way down to the ends. Now, blow-dry on cool for one minute and give your head a sexy va-va-voom, Brad-is-home-with-Chinese-takeout-and-I'm-half-naked-in-a-short-robe head toss. We can't promise any Brad will really show up, but you will definitely have sex kitten, full-body, hot hair.

AND ONE HAIR QUEEN WE'D LIKE TO MOVE IN WITH US (FOR INSPIRATION)

Primping problem du jour: You washed your hair yesterday and it's not dirty, and your stylist told you it's not good to wash every single day because it strips the natural oils from your hair. (Sad, but true.) But your hair is looking a little flat. Cindy Crawford says she'd go for the Velcro, as in rollers, but we'd like to give her tip a little twist. Put the Velcro rollers in, pop on a shower cap, and step into the shower. Just standing in the heat and the steam for a few minutes will cause your hair to take on the shape of the rollers, thus adding volume. It's a fine way to bump up your 'do in minutes. One more tip: Before taking out the rollers, blow-dry for a few seconds to really set the new look.

THE ROOTS OF THE MATTER

We've all seen the root touch-up kits that look like gigantic mascara wands. Yes, they'll get rid of your outgrowth, but often those kits make your hair stiff and hard to style. (So much for the color fix now that you're a matted-down mess.) But brilliant stylist Ken Pavés, who works with the Jessicas—Simpson and Alba—has a better solution for roots grown amok. He suggests spritzing some light hair spray onto the roots and then using certain eye shadows, including shimmering gold, as a quick fix for both blondes and light brunettes. Soft brown shadow is a quick trick to get rid of a few gray strands. Ken suggests his Pavés Professional Flawless Convertible-Proof Hair Spray, Yves Saint Laurent eye shadow in No. 9 Golden Radiance, and No. 10 Shimmering Brown as fabulous fix combos.

ROLL WITH IT BABY

It's Dax to the rescue. Trendy celebrity hot-spot salon Privé, which is the hair home to Madonna, Cameron Diaz, Britney Spears, Johnny Depp, Lucy Liu, Virginia Madsen, Christina Ricci, Daisy Fuentes, and Nicole Richie, has an amazing stylist named Dax, a man who sings the praises of hot rollers.

Not only does he use them, but his favorite brand is the cheapest one at Target! Dax is only happy to teach us mere hair mortals how to roll, set, and style like the stars.

In other words: Yes, Virginia (not Madsen), there is a wrong way to do a roll-up.

Here are a few of his tips:

- A good roll-up doesn't start with rollers. Dax says to brush your hair when it's dry, but comb it when it's wet. "You will keep the integrity of the hair," he promises. But Dax also cautions us to never brush our hair too much. "Brushing is only needed to distribute the oils in the scalp. It's best to do prior to washing."

- Cool it with the products. Dax says that less is more and too much will just weigh your hair down.

- You can roll while traveling. If you're traveling and don't want to bring your big bulky set of hot rollers with you, then throw in a few different sizes of Velcros. In fact, he says to pack them inside your sneakers or shoes if you're running out of room.

● If you have Asian hair: Do your blow-out first, but without a brush. Don't even brush while blowing out! Just use your fingertips! It makes a curl much easier later on.

● If you have African-American hair: It's most helpful to do a wet set, which means put the rollers in when your hair is damp, use a heavy-duty setting lotion, and then dry it.

● Hairy tidbit: Dax says to always make your appointment with your stylist the afternoon of your big event, but not too close to its actual start time. Your hair needs time to adapt both to you and to the weather outside. (Plus your stylist could be running *tres* late, which will up your stress and make your toes curl from the trauma of checking your pink, diamond-encrusted Michele watch three thousand times.) After you get your curl on or even your blow-out, don't brush your hair. No matter if you get caught by a stray wind or someone blows an air kiss too hard in your direction, resist the temptation to take out your brush! We can see you now! Put the brush down! You will only flatten your hair. You can make a few adjustments with your fingers, but don't go nuts. You will regret it. (Put that comb down, too. We can still see you.)

THE PROFESSIONAL ROLL-OUT ACCORDING TO DAX

Say a quick beauty prayer. (Dax didn't actually say that, but we think it can never hurt.)

- Get your rollers at Target or any beauty-supply place with the idea being the cheaper the better. Just invest in the right clips to hold the hot rollers in place. The white ones with the small teeth have the best grip.

- Start at the crown of the head and take hair into sections. Gently comb through. Make sure the hair section you're rolling up is no wider than the roller itself or it won't give you the curl.

- Before putting in the hot roller, spritz hair section with a light holding spray and comb it through, distributing it from root to ends. Pull the hair straight up from your head and make sure the ends are rolled up tightly and evenly.

- Don't be afraid to use different sizes of rollers to make a fun, dramatic look.

- Use bigger rollers on the sides, smaller around the face.

- Spin the curler as you are pulling it out. Spritz with holding spray all over very lightly and then shake sides, roots, and crown. Dax says you must shake it because brushing out your hot roller set will make you look too done-up and like you have cookie-cutter hair. And no one, we repeat, no one, wants to look like a cookie.

Food for Hair—Part One

Hi, honey. And we don't mean this as a come-on. Did you know that honey draws and traps moisture in your hair (while the leftovers taste pretty good on toast and in tea)? Mix one tablespoon of honey into your favorite shampoo. Rinse and watch your hair behave beautifully.

Rice makes your hair expand and look fuller. A trick is to put one cup of rice in two cups of water. Let this mixture sit. In the morning, put the resulting rice water in a spray bottle and mist your damp hair before you blow-dry. Your limp locks will be revived for pennies!

Meanwhile, apple cider vinegar is a perfect shine booster. Use a little bit of it after you shampoo and it will remove the build-up in your hair. We don't recommend this if you have color-treated hair.

Hip Hair Tip

We would like to inform you that hairstylists in the better salons in Germany tell their clients that one only applies deep conditioner to dry hair and never wet. Is this a *Wunderkunde* hair tip? Well, yes, because non-waterlogged hair strands actually soak in more of the product. The water seals your hair shaft and prevents the product from soaking in.

BB Extra: This is why before you jump into a chlorinated pool, always, always, always wet your hair down to seal the locks and prevent the chemical from getting in. As for conditioning your dry locks, remember that it's even better if you leave this in overnight and then rinse in the morning.

Food for Hair—Part Deux

If you're experiencing the type of oil that they don't find in Texas, there is a simple solution. Take five bags of mint tea, put them in your teapot, and brew. Cool off this mix and then shampoo. Pour the cooled tea over your head as a final rinse. Do this after your shampoo and conditioner are out. The mint acts as a natural astringent and gets rid of your oil slick.

WHO IS THAT MASKED WOMAN?

For a great and inexpensive hair mask to give you lush locks like Maggie Grace or Salma Hayek, just take an empty shampoo bottle and mix ½ cup dried rosemary with ½ cup of light olive oil. Let it sit and mingle overnight. Comb infused oil through dry hair and leave on for ten minutes. Wet hair, shampoo, and rinse out the drabbies.

CHAPTER 5

Strippers, Pole Dancers, and Carmen Electra

*I worked out all of the routines for **Dave**. He approved everything! I would come home from rehearsal and say, "Oh, honey, today we did the choreography for the lap dance." And he'd say, "Really! Do you want to try that out and see how it works?"*

—**Carmen Electra** on how she worked out routines for her strip dance exercise video on rocker Dave Navarro

It's hard enough to get my eyebrows waxed, let alone down there. And you will never see me in a bikini. That's one shot you will never see. Fugettaboutit. I never even got my ears pierced.

—**Oprah Winfrey** on why she will never get a Brazilian wax

It's about empowerment. It's about finding this place of comfort and confidence in your own body.

—**Teri Hatcher** on pole dancing as workout

I just accept them as a great accessory to every outfit.

—**Jennifer Love Hewitt** on her curves

This is our chapter rated R—for Racy. But let's face it. Kym is a married woman and Cindy has a fabulous relationship. We still think it's not fair for the strippers, Hollywood call girls, and pole dancers to have all the intimate beauty secrets. These should be for sexy women (and men) everywhere.

How do we compete with these hotter-than-hot ladies? It's easy. Just remember that he (or she) already loves you. Here are just a few tips to just push it over the edge and be your most desirable self.

TINTED LOVE

We know you're worrying about the Middle East, the national deficit, and last season's $670 Chloé four-inch wedges. Will they still be au courant come July? Not to add another fret to your worry platter, but now comes news that your nipple color might be standing between you and true happiness.

Stick with us here. Pinkie, from where else but Pinky's Palace in the San Fernando Valley, swears by this little beauty bombshell. She swears that she get better tips when her nipples look a soft shade of baby-doll pink. Pinkie ain't pink, but a bland flesh color in that area, which is why she concocted a cheap fix and a foolproof recipe. (A girl has got to be resourceful in this business.)

Pinkie grabs a touch of strawberry Jell-O powder and dabs a wet Q-tip in water. Then she gently paints the thin dye on her nipples. It's a natural, easy, quick, and safe fix for this sensitive area, and Pinkie has plenty of Benjamins (tips) in her G-string to prove it works. Now, we dare you to try that in your own bedroom. Of course, you can use the rest of the Jell-O as a low-fat dessert.

BREAST INTENTIONS

Savvy, a dancer on the strip in Vegas, says it's good to be plump and perky—and we're not talking about being a size 16 with a good personality. We're talking about breasts here. It can be a long shift at her club (or in any bedroom) and Savvy says it's hard to look excited—i.e., like you've just felt a cold chill in the chest area. All Vegas top-tip getters use this pole dancer secret: They grab their latest lip plumper! Many contain cayenne pepper and other ingredients that increase blood flow to the lips. Guess what? It does the same thing to nipples, making Savvy look excited. Ready for action? Try this at your own discretion.

BOOBS WITHOUT SURGERY

And just in case you want a boob job without the fuss and muss of going to the hospital and having a scary operation, may we suggest Takeouts? Packaged in an adorable pink Chinese takeout container, these are clean, natural-feeling silicone inserts that add a full cup size to what nature gave you. The costume designer on the remake of *The Stepford Wives* ordered fifty pairs, but no word if it was Nicole Kidman, Faith Hill, or Bette Midler who added a little bounce to her ounces. Kerry O'Brien of Her Look Enterprises says, "Women love Takeouts because they're a fun, functional and versatile fashion accessory. They can be worn with anything from a T-shirt to a tiara." If you're feeling too busy, you don't have to pull a Pamela Anderson and have a boob reduction surgery. Simply remove them from your bra when you want less shimmy in your shake. By the way, your pet boobs are washable with warm water and soap. Just keep them away from sharp objects because they will puncture. Get some cleavage at www.thebetterboobjob.com.

Now We're Blushing

Nars has a blush that's a flushed peachy color titled, what else, Orgasm. If you find it, buy it immediately because it's reportedly always out of stock at major department stores. By the way, there is also a matching lipstick and gloss that have sold out.

IMAGE MAKER: ALEXIS VOGEL

Pamela Anderson doesn't trust her ultrasexy face to anyone else. That would be flame-haired, ultrasexy-in-her-own-right makeup artist Alexis Vogel, who has perfected the bombshell, come hither, kitten look complete with the perfect pouty pucker for **Pammy**, **Paula Abdul**, **Sharon Stone Carmen Electra**, and **Gwen Stefani**, to name a few. *Playboy* even dubbed her their "secret weapon when it comes to makeup artists." If you want to vamp it up for the night, just continue reading and make sure your man has taken his heart medication.

What are your five favorite products in your bathroom right now?

- **Perfumia Gal Madrid Lip Balm**. I can't go to bed without it. I soak all of my clients' lips with this before I do their makeup, too. I've been using it for ten years now.

- **Lancôme Progrès Eye Crème**. It's been twenty years of using it. I love it and have to swear by this one. My under-eye area is still doing all right for my (cough, cough!) age! LOL!

- **Gillette Venus Razor for Women**. It's the closest shave you will ever get with a head that moves, and you will never get a cut or a nick. Shakira won't use anything else but this. I was on tour with her in Europe and she got me hooked! It's the best thing out there and shaves you so softly that it's unreal.

- **Alexis Signature Lip Gloss in Blitz**. I can't leave the house without my pouty lips on!

- **KMS Color Vitality Shampoo**. It's fantastic and smells so good. I've been using it since it came out. It's the best shampoo for dry or color-treated hair.

BUTT SERIOUSLY

Beverly Hills plastic surgeon Anthony Griffin argues that nothing says love on Valentine's Day like the gift of a Brazilian butt lift. "One guy bought this procedure for his girlfriend, who was in her 60s," he says. "The injections go deep into fat layers, sort of like Swiss cheese. We know from experience it lasts at least twenty years." Yes, A-list entertainers have had this done. It's nice because people can't really tell, and you can say you just really hit the Stairmaster. Top requested celeb butts include Beyoncé, Angelina, Tyra, and, of course, J.Lo.

SMELLS LIKE A HOT NIGHT

Christopher Gable makes perfect scents to us. He is the cofounder and genius behind Demeter Fragrances, the yummiest, sexiest, most coveted smells sweeping Hollywood and beyond. Jennifer Aniston reportedly used them in her Malibu home. Perhaps you've seen the little square bottles with the fab smells inside that can be used either on you or your house. (Cindy loves Fig while Kym is partial to Snow.) Other amazing ones include Sex on the Beach, Cosmopolitan, Cake Batter, Prickly Pear, Between the Sheets, and Dirt. They're so spot-on that you swear you smell the real thing.

At a chichi West Hollywood pre–Golden Globes soiree, Kym and Cindy asked Chris for his most startling news about smell. We had to sit down. "There is one scent that above all others turns men on. It even creates a . . . uh . . . physical reaction that proves they're excited," Chris tells us.

Yes, during the study it was cinnamon buns that actually caused men to have erections. "This was tested by a sensory institute and they've proven that cinnamon buns are the ultimate male turn-on," he adds. Now, what about the women? "The women got the most excited by pumpkin pie," he says. (Maybe that's because it's the only time we can have our pumpkin pie, but without calories and carbs, too! Any woman would find that stimulating!) Of course, Chris makes delish cinnamon and pumpkin pie scents.

Why are smells so important . . . and so sexy? Chris says, "Scent is so visceral. It touches our reptilian brain. There is even a nurse in Iowa who uses my Dirt scent with some of her Alzheimer's patients who were farmers."

What are Chris's favorites? "I do love Cinnamon Bun, of course, because I'm a man! I love our Dirt because it's very earthy but has a greenness that's very stimulating. You can't get much better than Vanilla Cake Batter." His suggestion for women who are looking to turn on their mates is pretty simple. "I like Gin & Tonic. It's uplifting. Manly. It's very seductive. I would also pick Vanilla Cake Batter because it's stimulating and comforting at the same time." So, we should spray Cake Batter on our inner thighs? "You should use the scents on different points of your body. Anywhere your guy likes . . . It can please his reptilian brain and his reptilian . . . other parts!"

BB Extra: If you don't have any Demeter on hand, you can use a dab of vanilla extract behind your ears to turn your guy on in that comforting way.

CANDIE'S CANDY

It's pretty obvious that strippers have to look good, thin, and extremely flat-tummied. Their livelihood depends on it. So one top Los Angeles exotic dancer, who goes by the name of Candie, gave us her tips. Let's just say she's as taut, tight, and thin as they come. And Candie says it's all due to her diet of candy, specifically jelly beans. She eats her beans, drinks lots of plain water, and also has been known to sip Red Bull. The drinks fill her up so she doesn't snack and she swears it helps her skin stay peachy. The jelly beans give Candie her energy for dancing and entertaining all night without the fat that is in other sweets.

BITE MARKS

Loved a bit too much? You can rub a dab of toothpaste over that hickey. Yes, we said the H word. There's nothing worse than a 45-year-old woman wearing a turtleneck in the middle of summer and sweating to death because her mate did some, uh, heavy necking. By the way, the toothpaste gets the red out and even speeds up the healing. You can also try a bit of concealer to hide the red spots.

BIKINI LINED

Even the best bikini wax can lose its smoothness a week later. What do you do about those unsightly ingrown hairs that are starting to drive you nuts? Well, first of all, leave them alone for the first twenty-four hours after you notice them so they can grow a little bit longer. Then get in the shower and get rid of them by gently going over them with a loofah. Remember never to pick at them. This will only make them worse and can even cause an infection!

BB Extra: **Pamela Anderson**, **Lisa Rinna**, and pole dancers get rid of razor bumps by using Tend Skin for ingrown hairs and razor burn. Put it on with a cotton ball after shaving and watch it work wonders.

STRIPPER BEAUTY SECRETS

In Hollywood, a pole has nothing to do with being proud of your Polish heritage. Pole people are those who have embraced a fitness craze known as pole dancing. Stars like Teri Hatcher and Carmen Electra plus some socialites insist that they love what this workout does for their bodies. But it turns out the admiration for this "lost art" goes a little deeper.

Even A-list types are looking to professional pole-dancing pros (Hollywood Beauty Speak: Your Strip Coach)—for a few beauty tips. You can't deny that these women look good day in and night out—focus on the nights. How do they do it without spending all their G-string money on pricey cosmetics?

We embarked on a little fact-finding mission (fully clothed) and found ourselves at a hot L.A. club where we met Amber, Summer, Cherry, Sissy, and (our favorite name) Paisley. (By the way, we hear that many A-list males have frequented the place, too, but we didn't see them on our visit—damn it all to hell!) We were mortified, however, to walk into the club only to feel the stare of the patrons. Remember, we had clothes on and didn't go near a pole! (We swear—especially if Kym's husband or Cindy's father has gotten this far in the book.)

Now, it's time to reveal the beauty secrets.

Amber told us that a girl just can't spend her tip money (oh no!) on expensive products. "Every night before I go to bed alone, which is not always, but when it happens, I smear on the old Neutrogena moisturizer and then I seal it with the cheapest beauty trick in the book. I put Vaseline right on top. Baby, my skin is as smooth as silk."

Summer summoned us into her dressing room to admit that her "natural" blonde "sun-kissed" hair gets a little bit of help when her roots start showing. "When I can't make it to the salon because I have a show or a date, I just grab an old toothbrush. You skirt on a dab of facial cream bleach. Brush it on your roots and you'll look luscious, honey! Listen to your friend Summer!"

Cherry gets her beautiful red hair to shine thanks to a quick trip to the grocery store. "I'm not one for muss and fuss," she says. "In fact, I buy whatever shampoo is on sale at Walgreens. But then to get my hair to glow in the dark—and I mostly work in the dark—I rinse with seltzer water. I use cherry. Get it!"

Sissy keeps her body smooth with the help of coconut oil. "Miss Things, my thing is I put large quantities of coconut oil lotion, which I buy at any drugstore, in my hair. It keeps it smooth and shiny for almost no money. It's perfect for women of color."

And finally, Paisley gave us two snaps and got out a bottle of deodorant. "I rub Sure deodorant, unscented, on my unmentionable area (enough said) right after shaving. I tell you, it's as smooth as a baby's . . ."

Thank you, ladies.

GLIDE INTO BEAUTY

Astroglide is known the world over as one of the top-selling personal lubricants. It's clear, smooth, silky, and it works . . . however, a few of our working-girl friends tell us that Astroglide has more than one use.

● Astroglide as a shaving cream. In the shower slather on legs, underarms (and whatever else you want to shave), and you will be silky smooth all over.

- Astroglide as a hair conditioner and frizz tamer. Just dab a small amount onto palm, rub hands together, and gently apply to hair. It smooths out frizz without weighing down the hair.

- Astroglide as a hand softener and skin conditioner. After putting on your fake tanner, wait for the color to dry and then rub onto skin. It helps to extend the life of the tan and works as a skin moisturizer.

- Astroglide is great for cuticles on fingers and toenails; it softens and nourishes skin.

Overheard on the Red Carpet: What A-list Hollywood legend *always* puts ice on her nipples before she shoots a scene because she mostly prefers to go braless and wear revealing, clinging clothing that leaves nothing to the imagination? Her dressing room requirements always include fresh flowers and a fully stocked ice bucket.

Tan Woman

We're glad you're using self-tanner instead of baking yourself in the sun, which is bad for both your skin and your heath. But now there's a new problem. Suddenly, you have the fabulous tanner on your palms and fingers and it's hard to get rid of that color where you don't want it. The solution is simple. Just cut a lemon in half and rub it on your skin where you want the tanner gone. You can also use a bit of salt. We promise that the color will be gone in an instant.

Under-Ruse

You're going to your own red-carpet event and you really need to look great, feel fabulous, and be the belle of the ball. Focus on your drawers. Venezuelans wear yellow underwear for good luck. They also write their wishes in a letter and burn it to make them come true. Hey, this is Hollywood and dreams really do come true. So, get out your yellow undies and a pen . . .

I, Spy

Whether they're strippers or socialites, exotic dancers or Malibu wives, ladies in the know always know that attraction starts with the most important beauty weapon: eye contact. A new study from Dartmouth College shows that a woman who can hold a man's gaze rather than averting her eyes is considered much more attractive and likable. So, get rid of your shyness and focus in like a laser beam. You are allowed to blink now and then so your eyes don't dry out.

BB Extra: What's a fast way to drop a quick five to ten pounds? An A-lister known for flaunting it told us the key is to put down your cocktail glass. She lost fifteen pounds in three months just by stopping social drinking, especially red wine and sweet drinks like cosmos that add tons of carbs to your daily diet. Another bonus is that once you stop drinking you're likely to also put down the junk food that most people mindlessly nibble on with their drinks.

ARE YOU CHILLY
OR JUST HAPPY TO SEE ME?

There's a famous mind-melting *Sex and the City* episode where Samantha pulls out a pair of fake nipples and insists they're the must-have fashion accessory. Let's nip this one right now: Some of us don't want to be walking sex on parade. What to do when you want to go braless but are mortified of walking into an air-conditioned room? Heather Locklear knows that you buy yourself some Low Beams: ouchless, latex-free teeny adhesive pads that you can wear with or without a bra. No way to put this delicately: You just slap these babies on your nipples and you're ready to go.

HOW TO LIVE LIKE A SEX KITTEN

We already told you that former *Playboy* makeup artist Alexis Vogel does the hottest hotties in Hollywood, from Pamela Anderson to Carmen Electra. She even gave Kelly Clarkson her steamy image for her new CD. We asked the sex kitten image maker how the average woman in Duluth, Minnesota, in temperatures twenty below zero with four kids and a limited budget can become her own sex kitten all the time?

Alexis suggests:

● It's all about the hair. Men love long, tousled, feminine hair. They don't have it, they want it, and they think it is sexy all the time.

● Start with the color. If your hair is dull, lifeless, and boring, then, for God's sake, go to the store and get some hair color and spice it up. Just go back to the color it used to be in high school. If it was blonder, go there. If it was a richer brunette, then go for that color again. If it was brighter red, then get busy. Make sure the color is rich and yummy.

● If your hair is short then "fem" it up! Make it hot-and-sexy short hair. The only tools you will need are a set of hot rollers. Use different sizes of the hot rollers. Alexis prefers Belson Profiles Spa P8329 set, which she uses on Pam, but any rollers will do. (It's just that these get very hot and so hold the curl for longer.) Take a small section of hair using the smaller hot rollers around the face line and then use the larger ones in the back. Before wrapping your hair, twist it in small sections and then mist with a protective spray. (Alexis likes Matrix Biolage Thermal-Active Setting Spray. It makes the hair soft.) Then wrap a roller around each twisted hair section and keep the rollers in while you perfume yourself, put on your makeup, step into your heels, and get dressed. Before you walk out the door, take out the rollers. DO NOT BRUSH OUT THE HAIR!!!!!! Tip your head upside down, massage scalp, tousle and spray *Waaaaa La!* You are the sex kitten supermodel of Duluth, or wherever you are!

● Don't forget your brows. Pencil them in or on just add some color with powder. Both will make you look more glamorous and sexy.

- If you are going to wear sweats out of the house, make sure they're colorful, soft, or pretty. Don't look like you just walked out of the gym after a long morning of doing cardio. In other words, no dead, gray, stinky, torn sweats in public!

- If you're a "My-Man's-T-Shirt-Only" girl then we're not going to get on your case. But you should know that a crewneck style cuts you off at the neck and adds weight to you while drawing attention to your chin area. A nice button-down neckline, on the other hand, elongates your neck and teases your admirers.

- Remember that Alexis says, "Celebrities are sexy creatures and sensual beings. They live it every day of their lives. They sleep on soft, high-thread-count, luxurious sheets even if they're sleeping alone. It's a soft, gentle way to soothe the skin." She says celebs always buy fresh flowers, filling vases throughout their homes with the scents of roses and beautiful colors while adding sensuality to the home. They also light candles all day long even if it's just to set a tone or a mood. It's about feeling good about yourself and your life. Just don't set the house on fire.

- Her biggest tip: Alexis wants to tell every woman out there, coast-to-coast, "Forget about the other woman. You have to *be* the other woman." She adds, "At all times have a bottle of wine chilled and ready at your home, because you never know. **Pam Anderson** always has a chilled bottle of expensive champagne in her fridge."

YOUR WISH IS OUR COMMANDO-MENT

We see London, we see France. On the red carpet, we do not want to see your underpants, even if they're $150 La Perla silky drawers. What's a starlet who abhors panty lines to do? Well, buy a Commando, a paper-thin undergarment that acts like a never-seen second skin. Jennifer Lopez swears by this product, which is made from a patented fabric (nah, they won't tell us nothin' about it). This low-rise thong-like treasure features no elastic, no trim, and thus no panty lines. But it's also so breezy to wear that it doesn't dig into your hips to the point where you feel like you're being prepped for lipo. We absolutely adore the colors you can buy: Tonight's the Night White, Birthday Suit, Buck Naked Nude, and Baby Got Back. And the sizes seem to cover all from a small (sizes 0 to 8) to a medium/large (sizes 8 to 14). Check out www.commandointimates.com.

Overheard on the Red Carpet: What Hollywood starlet, known for her fab figure, has recently put on a few pounds? Her chronically unemployed, Svengali-like husband is so interested in getting her body back that he controls her calories even when he's not around. Mrs. Thing went on a recent girls' night out and asked the waiter about dessert. "I'm sorry," the waiter implored. "I'm not even allowed to wheel the dessert cart over. Your husband called earlier today and threatened us. He also said that if any of your friends order dessert don't even bring it to them because you'll sneak a bite."

INTIMATE KNOWLEDGE

So you're running for the studio and the same bra you wore yesterday is dangling off the bathroom sink. Stop, put that lingerie down immediately, and take a gigantic step backward. You're saving a life . . . or the life of your $75 DKNY bra. A bra should never be worn two days in a row even if you just wore it for a few hours. Why? The elastic gets stretched out and stressed. And it seems that bras have needs, too. It takes them twenty-four hours for their elastic to recover from a wearing. By the way, it helps if you wash your bras in a net bag with cold water and then hang them to air dry.

BEAUTY IS PAIN (SOMETIMES)

Got razor burn? Ouch! Rub a lot of aloe vera gel over your legs before you shave so you won't burn those gams up. The gel also helps guarantee a close shave that will leave you hairless and silky smooth.

A CLOSE SHAVE

A quick tip if you're having any stubble trouble. You should always shave your legs in the morning instead of at night. Why? At the end of the day, your legs will be a teeny bit swollen so you'll never get a close shave.

Overheard on the Red Carpet: What Hollywood diva thought her hubby would be so upset when she downsized her DD breast implants to more tepid C cups that she went to their local jeweler and bought him a tiny bauble in the form of a ruby ring that cost her over $30,000? Word is hubby liked the ring but would have rather had the DDs in his life.

HOW TO WALK, TALK, AND CHEW IN YOUR MANOLOS

He's called the Sultan of Strut. Judge **J. Alexander** of *America's Next Top Model* was a runway model for Jean Paul Gaultier. His best red-carpet advice: Practice your prance. "It's best to put on heels as soon as you get them and get used to walking in them before you go out in front of the crowd," he advises. "That way you can walk the walk like you were born wearing stilettos." Also you should pay attention to your stance. In order to stand up completely straight, he says, imagine your body is an accordion from your midsection to your head. If you think about straightening out that section you will look thinner and your clothes will always look better.

IT'S HARD OUT HERE
FOR A POLE DANCER . . .

—A modified version of the 2006 Oscar-winning song

I pretend like I'm into him when I'm facing him. But when I turn around, I make faces at my friends and think about what I have to do the next day.

—Stacey, a top-ranking exotic dancer
at a high-class club in L.A.

And now we interrupt our regularly scheduled beauty tips for a few minutes of "Pole Talk."

It was all so civilized and intellectual. Kym met Miyoko, one of the top strip coaches and private pole-dancing instructors in town. She is a former actress, model, Playboy talk-show host (we didn't even know Playboy had talking) and the foremost expert on stripping, aka "strip coaching."

We met at a Calabasas, California, Barnes and Noble bookstore. Of course, the most demure-looking, glasses-touting, fully covered-up, Uggs-boots-wearing girl was Miyoko. It was a little embarrassing that Kym asked two nannies and a neighborhood salesgirl if they were the famous stripping coach Miyoko. All of them hissed at her and abruptly walked in the other direction. The shy, soft-spoken, Asian-American beauty simply smiled warmly and told Kym to sit down.

Okay, the interview definitely got started on the wrong Plexiglas high-heeled foot when Kym opened by nervously gushing, "Thanks so much for meeting with me. It's an honor to meet a real . . . strip coach, I mean . . . pole-dance instructor, and we will be sure to give you full exposure in the book!" (K: FULL EXPOSURE to a stripper! How tacky. I'm such a nonstripper interviewer.)

At that moment, our subject in question took the floor.

Miyoko: In pole dancing, many soccer moms and suburban housewives like yourself find a safe place to communicate feelings of resentment or neglect. I show everyday women how to beat the strippers, pole dancers, and lap dancers at their own game.

Kym: Miyoko, I don't want to sound like a total novice but . . . ummm . . . well, I am. So how do you start?

Miyoko: Well, its really just SPS—shower, primp, and shave. Put on some edible body dust to tempt his senses . . . my favorite is Kama Sutra Honey Dust . . . I dust it all over . . . ahhhhh and it smells and tastes great. Also don't forget about the details . . .

Kym: Ummmm, you don't have to get *too* detail-oriented. (I squirmed, noticing a few strange men hanging out near our table.)

Miyoko: By details, I mean, paint your toenails. Toes and feet can be incredibly sexy. It's not really just for him. You'll notice an added boost of self-esteem by spoiling your piggies with some pampering. Here's another tip: Go either extreme like fire-engine red or nude soft pinks—most men don't like the in-between colors . . . Now, let's talk tooooools. . . .

Kym: (Adjusting my pen and paper nervously) No, no, no . . . we really don't have to hear about your favorite toys and electric . . .

Miyoko: (Purring) I didn't say toys. I said "tools," as in personal hygiene. Lashes, there's something about them—you just feel and look more sexy. Most exotic dancers have battled with ingrown hairs and razor burn from shaving so often (basically every day). Skin Tend is the only answer. The Mach 3 razor had been all pole dancers' number-one choice for years. Now, it's the Fusion with five blades. It gets really close, especially if you use lots and lots of shaving cream. Ohhhhh, and you can also use the shaving cream . . .

Kym: Never mind, Miyoko. Let's stick with the hygiene tips.

Miyoko: Nair is also an insider, if you know what I mean, trick of the trade.

Kym: [I didn't dare ask for details. Some things are better left to the imagination!]

Miyoko: (Meowing now) Ohhh, here's another tip. Lighting is everything. Strippers have an amazing aura of angelic performance when onstage and it's not because they are angels." (She said it, I didn't.) You won't feel particularly sexy if you are obsessing over every little butt zit or razor bump, so let's keep those lights to a minimum. Get a low-watt bulb in your bedroom lamp and change it right before you head for bed. Stage yourself ladies. The other girls do it!

Kym: How can you make yourself seductive even if you're not J.Lo?

Miyoko: Men look at women's bodies in pieces. If you present to them what you want them to see, then that's what they will look at! The best strippers, dancers, and adult performers master communicating. They're telling a story and drawing attention to the parts of the body they feel the best about and want to draw attention to.

Kym: What do women do beauty-wise that's a turn-off to men?

Miyoko: Women wear too much perfume and too much make up!!! [She hissed this as she looked directly at me with her scrubbed-clean, makeupless face and flawless skin.] Your own body scent is much more primal to him than splashing on tons of synthetic chemicals.

Kym: What has been your most extreme or expensive purchase for beauty, dancing, or teaching?

Miyoko: Laser!!!! So worth it. We in the biz call it "fully landscaped." [Enough said.]

Kym: What is your favorite inexpensive beauty tip or product to use before pole dancing or stripping?

Miyoko: Blush stain and a bubble bath . . .

Kym: [Blush stain and bubble bath, now you're talkin' my language, sista. Getting a little confident, I started to think maybe I *was* a future pole dancer in the making! That visual came to a screeching halt when Miyoko started extolling the secrets of the real top-ranking dancers. Staring right into my eyes, she confidently purred . . .]

Miyoko: Penetrate men with your gaze. Most dancers will tell you, "If you can look a guy in the face and stare him down, you've got him."

Kim: Really, Miyoko? With all due respect, the last time I did that was in third grade with Steve Toldy during a staring contest. After less than two minutes, I got bored and walked away, forfeiting the grand prize of an old, stale Tootsie Roll.

Miyoko: Exactly! It's just like playing a game in elementary school!

It was actually her last statement that was the most intriguing to me. Miyoko confessed that her best striptease was wearing a pair of sweats for her husband of six years. With her smooth, clean skin and naturally flat chest, the performer said, "The average woman gets too much surgical modification—the fake boobs, the daytime porno makeup, the latest fashion trend, whether it looks good on her body or not. It's all too much, and inside they have nothing *real* to communicate."

"You know," she whispered, "when I was working at a very high-class private L.A. club, the girls that were requested all the time and got the biggest tips were not necessarily the most beautiful. They were the most confident. They knew how to carry themselves. They had self-acceptance and self-love. At the time, I was envious of it. Now I've developed it for myself and here's the biggest news: You can't learn it!"

BB Extra: According to top-rated strip coach **Miyoko,** "One thing strippers and call girls know that the other women don't is that men like variety. Ladies, if you can create that for them at home, they don't have to go anywhere else. One night be a little more **Beyoncé**, another night take on **Mariah**'s style. Find a persona in yourself that wants to come out!"

CHAPTER 6

Over 40 and Fabulous!

I do care what other people think. I have my issues with my looks. But I feel if I frame it right, I'll look just a little bit better than what I was given.

—**Diane Keaton**

I'm not 20. Not 30. But I'm certainly different from what most people feel someone in her 40s should be.

—**Demi Moore**

Not to be cliché, but there really is something about turning 40. I've quit defining myself by what I'm not, and I'm thinking about what I am.

—**Teri Hatcher**

You have to start by changing the story you tell yourself about getting older. If you're telling yourself a story about what you're losing and fear, then that's just the story you're going to live. You've just cast yourself in a plot. So the minute you say to yourself, "Time is everything, and I'm going to make sure that time is used the way I dream it should be used," then you've got a whole different story.

—**Diane Sawyer**

I'm the same person. I've just grown to be more of myself with better shoes.

—Oprah Winfrey

Laughter! That's what the invincible Sharon Stone says is her secret to looking young. That is seriously funny to us. We also love the one from the University of Texas at Austin. Yes, a university study determined that people in their 40s are more secure and relaxed than those who are younger. That sounds lovely, except we can't possibly relax unless we have the best beauty tips that will truly make us secure in our 40s. The truth is we do want to look a few years younger. And who really wants to relax that much? Read on . . .

TÉA FOR YOU!

There are few women we love more than Téa Leoni. She looks effortlessly gorgeous with almost no makeup on while acting and mothering her two beautiful kids with equally amazing husband David Duchovny.

Cindy spent more than a few minutes with Téa at the Waldorf-Astoria Hotel in New York City on a freezing winter day, but the beauty tips warmed everyone up.

A HOLLYWOOD BEAUTY MOMENT
WITH TÉA

Cindy: Téa, you always look fabulous, but effortlessly so. Plus you have a perfectly thin, but not anorexic, body. Should we hate you? Should we weep? And while you're at it, what are your best beauty tips?

Téa: I used to work out for my ass, but now I work out for my heart. But I think the ass is still benefiting. I wear a lot of sunscreen. I think that helps, and also drinking water. I also love to walk and do Pilates. And please don't hate me. I struggle with it just like you do.

Cindy: We could never hate you, especially now that we've heard that you're really anti-Botox. What do you have against that little needle?

Téa: Please say no to Botox. I'm really against cosmetic work. Don't get me wrong. I'm dying to do it. But it makes me feel bad. It's this idea that we have to do it. I'm 40 and I feel the sexiest I've ever felt. I'm better in bed. I'm smarter. I have children and the lines that come with it. You can see my life in my face. My lines say that I've been laughing a lot and that's a beautiful thing. I hate the idea of the woman who earned those lines making them go away with a shot or a scalpel. I want the lines to say, "Congratulations you're better than when you were 23 and had no lines."

Cindy: Don't you have a funny deal with actress Elisabeth Shue?

Téa: Liz Shue and I have a pact. If we flirt with a Botox needle, we'll call each other and stage an intervention.

Cindy: Do you really feel better now? Or are you just saying that because I just turned 40 and need an intervention?

Téa: You don't need an intervention! I do think back to my 20s. I was a little hottie back then, but things change. I'm still hot, but now I have a life. And I'm looking forward to being 60. Can you imagine how smart I'll be then, lines and all?

40 AND FAB—A PRIMER!

Okay, you don't have to be 20 to be gorgeous. We culled the best beauty tips for those 40 and beyond:

● Hollywood makeup gurus insist that less is more when you hit 40. The first thing to lighten up on is your eyeliner. Forget black and opt for a softer brown or even a gray.

● Exchange dark lip pencils for nude. Nude pencils create a younger look and prevent your lipstick from running north or south. Dust a little translucent powder over your lipstick to set the look, or just use a bit of shimmering lip gloss over the liner instead. By the way, forget pink lipstick if your teeth aren't shiny white. It'll make your teeth look yellow.

- Make sure to fill in your brows with powder rather than pencil. The powder will last the entire day, and will erase five years from your face.

- To hide a little extra skin hanging from your jawline, contour with a powder that's one or two shades darker than your natural skin. Start at the front of your chin and work it along your jaw for an instant pick-me-up.

- We know you know, but for the sake of all that is holy and gorgeous, stay out of the sun and use sunscreen if you must step outdoors.

- Drink water.

- To make your eyes look wide again, use eyeliner on your top lashes followed only by an application of mascara. Go for thicker mascara on the outer corners of your eyes to make them look ten years younger.

- If you have brown or black hair, see gray hairs popping through, and can't get to the salon, grab some mascara. It gets rid of the gray in two seconds.

- Exercise, but don't kill yourself. Sophia Loren says that she simply walks about an hour a day. Susan Sarandon relies on Pilates.

- Sleep. Sophia also hits her pillow by nine each night to let her body repair itself while she sleeps. Silk pillowcases decrease your chances of getting fine lines.

- Pack on about five pounds. If your face looks saggy and harsh, a little bit of weight can make it look like you've had a major lift. Salma Hayek, 40, just put on ten pounds. "I like to look a little bit curvier and my face looks great," she says. "I also had fun eating a few burgers and fries."

- Get rid of the frosted eye shadows and opt for matte or warm tones. This deeper, richer look will erase years.

- Whiten your teeth. As you get older they become more porous and discolor more easily. A good smile can make your age fade into the sunset.

- Stop smoking. Your lungs can't take it, it robs your skin of oxygen, it creates tons of fine lines around your lips, and it makes your teeth look a garish yellow. Did we mention your poor lungs?

- Wear some fab Chanel sunglasses. They look great, and they'll stop you from squinting, preventing the formation of fine lines.

- Forget the salt. It will make your eyes look puffier after age 30.

- Take vitamins A, B complex, C, E, and minerals and zinc. Each helps to repair your skin while you sleep. A pretty good deal, if you ask us.

A WONDERFUL WOMAN

We checked in with Lynda Carter, the eternal beauty who played Wonder Woman, and she didn't deflect our questions with her magic gold bracelets (even then she knew bangle bracelets were cool).

"I've always been a soap and water girl," Lynda tells us. "Forget the expensive stuff. Just give me a bar of Neutrogena soap and a washcloth."

"Every couple of weeks, I'll do an egg-white mask," she adds. "I love how people make masks sound so complicated. I grew up in Phoenix and my mother was always on me about my skin. She would say, 'Lynda, do you want to grow up with a face that looks like a lizard purse?' So, I always wear a hat when I go outside in the summer and I never leave the house without sunscreen on my face, neck, and hands."

BB Extra: Lynda says, "Keep some sunscreen in your car and put it on your hands when you drive. A few years ago, I noticed I was getting those ugly brown spots on my hands. Then I figured out that I drive so much that my hands were getting exposed to the sun while I held the steering wheel. So, keep a high SPF sunscreen in the car and cream your hands so they're not exposed. It's also great to remember to put it on your neck, so you won't feel like you're 8,000 years old."

BETWEEN A SHARON STONE
AND A HARD PLACE

Sharon Stone. We're taking a Pepcid just thinking about her fabulous new look. La Stone won't give up too many secrets about how she stays looking sooo young as she approaches the big 5-0, but after extensive research, *The Black Book* has uncovered a few tips we could all learn from: Sharon's confidence about her fashion sense makes her look beautiful. She even gives herself haircuts. (Now, that *is* confidence.) She owes her lean, thin bod and always-flat tummy not to exercise (which she claims she hates), but to cutting out sweets and between-meal snacks.

AGE ERASERS

According to stylist Ricci DeMartino, who has worked with Courtney Cox Arquette, Helen Hunt, and Lisa Kudrow, there is a trick that the stars use to show over-40 arms at their best when being photographed. Simply pose for pictures with your hands on your hips, elbows pointed back. You've just trimmed your arms in the photo by many inches.

CELE-BEAUTY: JANE SEYMOUR

There are many over 50 who won't see eyelash-to-eyelash with former Bond girl and *Dr. Quinn* star Jane Seymour. The perennial screen beauty insists that she doesn't get her lifetime gorgeous cred with knives or shots.

"No Botox. No face-lifts," Jane tells *The Black Book*. "No obsessive running. No private trainers. None of that nonsense!" So what is Seymour saying "yes" to these days, because obviously it's working? "I'll tell you what makes me beautiful. A number of years ago I nearly died. I was very sick and in the hospital. I actually left my body," she says. "At that moment I realized that you take nothing with you including your perfectly smooth, line-free face. All you really have in this life is how you feel and what you're going to leave behind." Thank goodness, Jane recovered from her illness, but she says that epiphany gave her a new lease on life. "Life is not about getting beauty treatments, but about my kids, my husband, and the relationships I have with people. The happiness of concentrating on those things makes me feel beautiful."

A MOMENT WITH DIANE LANE

BB: What is the secret of looking so great after 40?

Diane: I think it's that I smile a lot. I think anyone who smiles automatically looks better. Try it at home.

BB: Do you have some exercise regime besides flashing those pearly whites?

Diane: I prefer yoga although it's the hot thing right now. It's a good thing to have so much yoga in the world. They say you are the age and the flexibility of your spine. If your spine is youthful and limber then you too shall be in other departments in your life. Flexibility is more important to me than strength or stamina. You have to be flexible in this life.

CELE-BEAUTY: VANNA WHITE

We don't have to spin the wheel to get the letters to spell out that Vanna White is B-E-A-U-T-I-F-U-L. She began hosting *Wheel of Fortune* in 1982 as the chief letter-turner and has hardly changed a bit. A full-time mom to two children, Vanna is one of the most down-to-earth women in Hollywood. She's known for wearing jeans and no makeup.

What is a high-end, over-the-top expensive, just-can't-live-without purchase for beauty you've made and why does it work so well for you?

La Mer. Because my skin loves it.

What is your favorite inexpensive or homemade beauty tip or product?

When I get a big pimple on my face, I put 100 percent pure alcohol on a Q-tip and dab it right on the pimple! It dries it up or brings it to a head quickly.

What does your beauty routine consist of on a daily and nightly basis?

I wash my face with a washcloth and Estée Lauder's Splash Away in the morning and before bed. Once a week, usually on Sundays, I give myself a quick facial with Estée Lauder's DermSolutions Refinish and Protect.

What are your all-time, never-fail, top-five best beauty products?

Moisturizer, under-eye concealer, eyelash curler, mascara, Lip Smackers lip balm.

If you were going to your own private island and could take only a limited beauty "stash," what would it be?

I'd take Estée Lauder's DermSolutions Refinish and Protect.

What is your secret antiaging tip?

Drink lots of water, eat right, and exercise. Boring, but true.

Give us your favorite health and diet tip.

Only eat when you're hungry. It's hard to do, but once you learn to listen to your stomach, you will find we eat more than we should. For example, entrées at a restaurant are huge. You don't need all that food on your plate. I usually share an entrée with someone when I go out to dinner. It's plenty!

What do you do a month before, a week before, and the day of a big event to make sure you look your best?

I follow a regular exercise routine throughout the whole year whether we are taping or not. It's six days a week. I usually spin for forty-five minutes, five days a week and also run on a treadmill three days a week for a mile or two before spinning. Then I do push-ups, sit-ups, and side bends.

BUTT SERIOUSLY

No, we are not calling you names. It's just that butts are BIG business in Hollywood, and although everyone's got one, everyone wants a bigger, tighter, and smoother one than the person next to them, especially if that person is J.Lo. This leads us to our next expert: Octavia of the Jim Wayne Salon in Beverly Hills, who is now on our speed dial. Her clients include Mischa Barton, Katie Holmes, and Nicollette Sheridan.

Octavia says she wouldn't think of leaving her house each morning without slathering on her must-have product, Butt-Firming Cream. "It smoothes out the derriere and keeps you toned and lifted. It's amazing and I can't live without it," says the facialist.

Speaking of junk in the trunk, celebrity moms swear by A + D Ointment, a heavy-duty cream made to help ease the pain of irritating diaper rash on babies' bottoms. These resourceful babes say it is one of the best moisturizers for hands, feet, and elbows!

And as a final footnote, the sales reps at Frederick's of Hollywood tell us they still can't keep the padded Butt Panties in the store ever since J.Lo made much of the world see that when it comes to your backside, bigger is better.

THE GOOD DOC IS IN

Top Santa Monica plastic surgeon Dr. Patrick Abergel caters to supermodels, actors, and actresses in L.A. and has been dubbed "a real-life ER doc" because of his charming, suave good looks. He's a member of the American Boards of Cosmetic Surgery, Laser Surgery and Dermatology, and to top it all off, he's French.

In most cases, Abergel says if you want to look younger and are over 40, focus on your eyes. He suggests his twenty-minute laser surgery to get rid of bags with no downtime, and you're back to work the next day. Another insider secret is that many Hollywood actresses who are approaching 40 see Dr. Abergel to smooth out the crinkly tissue most of us get on our eyelids after the age of 25. He uses another laser to "vaporize" the top layer of skin.

He says a woman should start seeing a plastic surgeon when she starts seeing flaws. "Correct the little things before they become big things," he says.

What doesn't work? He's not a big fan of the trendy new "thread lifts" where you lift up the sagging skin with thread. He also doesn't like thermage, a nonsurgical, muscle-stimulating lift for the face and neck. "If you want to look younger, forget those techniques and go for a mini-lift that will eliminate the jowls," he says.

What is a far less expensive and intrusive way to look glowing and young? Dr. A says there is an old French beauty secret he was taught long ago by a French doctor. French? Secret? Doctor? We're all ears.

"Take some cold milk, which is a protein, and pour it onto a washcloth, lay it on your face for a few minutes, and rest. Then switch to a warm compress of a washcloth soaked in hot tea because of its antioxidant properties," says the doc. "The alternating from cold to warm, protein to antioxidants, will increase blood flow to the skin and give you a glow that costs practically nothing."

BB Extra: Dr. A says one of the worst things you can do for your skin is to smoke. Smoking promotes aging and stops oxygen from being delivered to the skin. Sugar puffs you up, and soda "changes the structure of fat in your skin," says Dr. A. In other words, hello cellulite! He calls his eating regime for perfect skin Green, Green, Broil. At each meal, eat a green salad, a green veggie, and a broiled piece of fish or lean protein. One of the best things you can do for your skin post-40 is thirty to forty minutes of cardio a day.

Overheard on the Red Carpet: What over-40-year-old (almost 50) blonde bombshell tells all the press and interviewers that she never exercises and is just naturally thin (giggle, giggle) and sexy from loving life and being happy? However, insiders reveal that the star just purchased an at-home, cellulite-be-gone machine called a Wellbox for over $1,750 to work on the dimples on her bum. Oh, she probably doesn't have any (nobody in Hollywood does—uh-huh), but it is insurance for the bottom line . . . down the line.

CELE-BEAUTIES: JILLIAN BARBERIE AND DOROTHY LUCEY, ANCHORS, *GOOD DAY L.A.*

Kym has worked on Los Angeles's number-one-rated morning show *Good Day L.A.* on Fox for over eight years. The female anchors are two of her favorites in the business because they don't take the business, their reports, or, most important, themselves too seriously. They are gorgeous, successful women who have stood the test of time.

Dorothy is in her 40s and Jillian is about to hit 40, and they are both fabulous. Jillian is one busy woman, rising day in and day out, for more than ten years, at 3:30 in the morning. Her prize is coming into the studio and eating egg whites. Dorothy has a young son and a news reporter husband. She's at the studio by 4:00 in the morning and has to drive in from her home in tony Malibu. Dorothy shuns egg whites and eats oatmeal for breakfast. Dorothy works out and runs or does cardio every day, while Jillian hasn't done an exercise since she was 14 (which she will proudly tell you!). She doesn't even count her recent stint on *Skating with the Stars* as cardio.

These two may be as different in their routines and looks as night and day, but they share one thing in common: They've stayed on top in Tinseltown, a place where at age 23 you're usually pretty much put out to pasture as a newscaster. Yet, these two show up, do their jobs brilliantly, and shine.

Here are a few of their tips for staying powerful, sexy and beautiful day in and day out . . .

CELE-BEAUTY: JILLIAN BARBERIE

What are your high-end, over-the-top expensive, just-can't-live-without purchases for beauty?

Hair extensions and spray tan. I can't live without them and do both often.

What is your favorite inexpensive or homemade beauty tip?

Jurlique Pure Rosewater Freshener Spray.

BB Extra: Many of our favorite celebs, like **Gwyneth Paltrow** and **Madonna**, use this organic skin-care line. **Jillian**'s skin is flawless, and she wears heavy makeup under hot lights every day of the week, so it must work!

What does your beauty routine consist of on a daily and nightly basis?

I use Continuously Clear facial wash, vitamin A, and Serious Skin Care.

What are your all-time, never-fail, top-five best beauty products that you can't live without?

Lancôme Tinted Moisturizer
Dr. Brandt Lineless Eye Cream
Continuously Clear Moisturizer, with salicylic acid
Laboratoire Remède Photo Close-up under base moisturizer
MAC Strobe Cream

What is your secret antiaging tip?

Sunscreen, water, and sleep.

What do you carry in your teeny evening bag for a quick touch-up at red carpet events?

Breath mints and lip gloss!

How did you get those killer abs?

Low-carb diet and Vitamin Water, but I ate major carbs while I was skating and training.

What do you do a month before, a week before, and the day of a major event to make sure you look your very best?

I sleep and stay away from "Big, Major Events."

Give us a beauty tip you do when traveling on your private plane or to a friend's manse or to a faraway location.

Ambien, water, and my facial mist (the Jurlique Rosewater spray).

Who do you think is the most beautiful woman in the world?

Kate Moss and Halle Berry.

What is the craziest thing you've ever done for beauty?

Electrolysis. Ouccccccch! And laser hair removal.

What is a secret beauty tip you share only with close friends?

Make love to a handsome man before a big event. It will give you the best glow!

Finish this sentence: I feel red-carpet ready when . . .
I wear Dolce and Gabbana.

What toothpaste do you use, favorite hair products, perfume, jeans . . .

I'm old school. I use Crest toothpaste. I love Kérastase hair products, Hanae Mori perfume, and True Religion jeans.

What is your in-a-quick-pinch, at-home beauty fix?
I do an enzyme face mask and take a long, hot bath.

What is your most unusual beauty tip?
I put crushed avocados on my face and take oatmeal baths.
I also use Korean washcloths to exfoliate my body.

BB Extra: Korean washcloths are inexpensive, softer, and create less tearing on your face. Allegedly, **Cindy Crawford** has been to Korea, washcloth-wise, if you know what we mean.

CELE-BEAUTY: DOROTHY LUCEY

She often refers to herself as a semireformed gossip reporter. Morning show host Dorothy Lucey works at the hot *Good Day L.A.*, a fun-filled, three-hour news and celebrity bonanza. "It's three hours packed with crap. Sorry, Mom. She hates when I use less than ladylike words!" Dorothy tells us. (We love an anchor with a sense of humor.) Yes, she hosts a news show, but most of the news seems to be about Britney and Brangelina. "Since I get made up at 5:00 in the morning, my face is usually asleep and very puffy," Dorothy says. "In fact, I often resemble a puffer fish. My whole beauty goal is to take away the puffiness. . . . Perhaps if I stopped eating chips and drinking wine before bed that would help. But since that will never happen, most of my beauty tips are of the antiaging, antipuffy variety. Enjoy!"

What is a high-end, just-can't-live-without beauty purchase and why does it work so well for you?

To counteract all the before-mentioned chips, wine, and don't forget candy, I take vitamins. As you can see, I'm such a health nut. If you catch me eating a vegetable it's to impress my 7-year-old son. Every morning I take a packet of Dr. Perricone's Skin & Total Body Nutritional Supplements. There are eight pills per packet, so it's a bunch to get down. But it forces you to also drink tons of water, which is also good to get things going in the morning. By the way, Dr. P is available online so you can have it sent to you.

What is your favorite inexpensive or homemade beauty tip or product?

My favorite drugstore products are Neutrogena. They're (relatively) cheap and they work. I use the Visibly Firm Lift Serum and the Visibly Firm Face Lotion every morning.

What does your beauty routine consist of on a daily and nightly basis?

In the morning (at 4:30 A.M.—aren't you sad for me?), I take my vitamins. I use the face serum and lotion and my eye cream. Right now, I'm using Dr. Wu's (Dr. Jessica Wu in L.A. She is a fabulous doctor to the stars and wannabes like me) White Peony Eye Contour Cream. Here's the best tip I stole from Dr. Wu: Keep the cream in the fridge. It acts like an ice pack and helps with puffy morning eyes. After the show, I wash off all of the icky sticky makeup, except my eyes, especially if my wonderful makeup artist has put on false eyelashes. It makes my mommy friends laugh when we go for a hike and I have lashes out to my elbows. I usually forget I have them on unless they hit my sunglasses. I leave the eye makeup on so my face doesn't feel naked. I also use a tinted sunscreen on my face. Stila makes a nice one, and if I'm feeling creative, I will mix it with the Revlon Skinlights. At night, I wash off all the TV makeup and sunscreen and use Neutrogena.

What are your all-time, never-fail, top-five best beauty products that you simply can't live without?

Number one is Dr. Perricone's Alpha Lipoic Acid Lip Plumper. It helps with those lines around the lips. I think we get lines from puckering up . . . to water bottles! Number two is Neutrogena lip gloss. I like any of the light pinks. I call pink my no-face-lift color. It always makes you look younger. Number three is the Philosophy Oxygen Peel. Three minutes and your skin feels like a baby's you-know-what. Four is vitamins. Five is keep whatever eye cream you use nice and cold.

If you were going to your own private island and could only take a limited amount of beauty and skin-care products what would you pack?

If I had to pick a luxury item (or two) for *Survivor*, I'd take my tinted sunscreen and lip gloss.

What is your secret antiaging tip?

Stay out of the sun (of course). I learned that one about thirty years too late. Since my little boy is such a beach baby, I often wear a cowboy hat. It saves the skin and you don't even have to comb your hair.

Give us your favorite diet tip.

I love coffee, but when I stopped hitting Starbucks three times a day, I started to lose weight. Now I try to drink mint tea. It's yummy. It's not a latte. But it's still good. Vitamins also keep me alive.

What do you do a month before, a week before, and the day of a big event to make sure you look your very best?

Once a week, I do the oxygen peel. Other than that I'm pretty lazy.

What is the most unusual item you've used in the name of beauty?

I've used toothpaste to kill a zit. I think tea tree oil works better, but toothpaste comes in handy.

Finish this sentence: I feel red-carpet ready when . . .

I feel red-carpet ready when I make sure my bra straps aren't showing. At the Emmys one year I was interviewing Joan Rivers. I had the dress, the hair, and the bra strap. Here I was thinking, "Joan, even you must think I look amazing." And when I looked at the video all I could see was the strap!

What toothpaste do you use, conditioner, shampoo, perfume, favorite designer jeans . . .

I use whatever toothpaste my husband buys. He always seems to be the one who stops at the drugstore. I like John Frieda Sheer Blonde Honey to Caramel Shampoo and Conditioner. The Alterna White Truffle Shampoo is nice as a treat, but it's expensive. I wear Micheal Kors perfume.

My jeans are whatever ones I can get my ass into that day. I like Hudson, Serfontaine, and even Gap. I also wear Da-Nang pants because they feel like sweats.

What is your favorite at-home, in-a-quick-pinch remedy for beautiful hair?

A little apple cider vinegar gives hair a nice shine, but you will smell like a salad.

IMAGE MAKER: IRENA MEDAVOY

A note from Kym: I met Irena Medavoy when our little boys were just born. She is a true California beauty—six feet tall; long, silky blonde hair; big crystal-blue eyes. She won't tell you this, but she was a model and actress before meeting her husband, Mike Medavoy, a former movie studio chief and now head of Phoenix Pictures. He has spearheaded numerous Oscar-winning films and together they are Hollywood royalty. Let's put it this way . . . whenever Irena walks into a room, all heads turn.

A note from Irena: "I'm a 47-year-old charity executive, writer, wife, and proud mother of an 8-year-old boy named Nicky. I'm also a founding board member of Team Safe-T and coach for kids' charities. I'm trying to pass a law in California to give patients the right to full disclosure on doctors' relationships with the drug companies. Before a doctor prescribes a drug or treatment for you, you must know if he is getting money from that drug company to promote that use.

"Since I'm unable to use Botox, collagen, or any fillers, I must rely very heavily on my skin products. They're all I have to keep looking my best, and they must work for my skin type."

What is a high-end, over-the-top expensive, just-can't-live-without purchase for beauty you've made and why does it work so well for you?
Crème de la Mer mixed with Ole Henriksen Lavender Creme. The two together at night make my face look better in the morning, which is a miracle.

What is your favorite inexpensive or homemade beauty tip or product?
The Body Shop Camomile Gentle Eye Makeup Remover is inexpensive and works better than any other brand. Plain yogurt as a face mask. Aquaphor for dry skin.

What does your beauty routine consist of on a daily and nightly basis?
I always take off all makeup at night, even on a plane.

What are your all-time, never-fail, top-five best beauty products that you can't live without?
Ole Henriksen On the Go Exhilarating Cleanser
La Mer and Ole Henriksen Lavender Creme on the face
Ole Henriksen Fresh Start Eye Creme
Body Shop Camomile Gentle Eye Makeup Remover
Clarins Instant Smooth Perfecting Touch

If you were going to your own private island and could take only a limited amount of beauty and skin-care products, what would they be?

Chantecaille Future Skin Foundation in cream or nude
Carmex lip ointment
Banana Boat aloe moisturizing body treatment
Lancôme black mascara
Serious Skin Care Dry-Lo

What is your secret antiaging tip?
Sex and the south of France. Sex in the south of France, even better.

Give us your favorite health or diet tip.
POM juice. I believe in pomegranate juice for health and beauty along with that plain yogurt secret that my Russian grandmother taught me. After all, just take a look at all of the Slavic models in the fashion magazines. They were weaned on old-fashioned plain yogurt. European diet. Drink, eat, just in moderation. Enjoy life and it will reflect on your face.

What do you do a month before, a week before, and the day of a big event to look your very best?
Swim. I love to swim all year long. It is my favorite exercise, and before an event I try to get in as much swimming and sleep as possible the night before.

Tell us about the biggest beauty blunder you see on other women.
Over-lipped, over-botoxed, over-fat-injected. Has anyone ever seen that kind of face in nature or in art? Because it never existed until some doctor sold the idea of "enhanced beauty" that has crossed over every threshold of natural.

And then the woman looks like every other woman from the same plastic tribe. Know when to stop. A little is one thing, gross exaggeration is ugly.

What is the wackiest thing you've ever done for beauty?
When I was 3 years old, I wanted to look like my beautiful blonde mother. We were painting the house, and there was a can of yellow paint. I stuck my long hair in it and my scalp felt like it was on fire. A trip to the ER and turpentine cured hair-dyeing for a while. Now I leave it up to Negin Zand, a color genius.

What is one beauty tip you share only with your closest friends?
Ardell individual lashes at $4.00 a kit. Just glue a couple on the outside of your eye, and it's the sexiest you can look. Or go to Marlena Fields at Umberto, who does the best eyebrows and individual eyelash makeup application in Los Angeles.

Finish this sentence: I feel red-carpet ready when . . .
I feel red-carpet ready when my son whistles at me.

What toothpaste do you use, conditioner, shampoo, jeans, perfume . . .
Colgate toothpaste, Terax hair conditioner, Kérastase green shampoo, Caroline Herrera is the *only* perfume I use. Listerine Orange mouthwash. Designers—Ralph Lauren, Dior, Valentino, Escada, Kira Craft, and Senso. Jeans—7 For All Mankind, and Martin Katz jewelry.

What is something you do to make yourself feel beautiful?

I put rose petals in my bra. My grandmother told me to do it.

Who do you think is the most beautiful woman in the world and why?

My mother, Rita Gerasimenko. She looked like a young Ingrid Bergman, stylish, classic, natural, and sexy. I loved her style, big glasses, wavy blonde hair, European accessories, and completely natural God-given gifts. She is my inspiration, was and will always be when it comes to aging gracefully. She said to always make the best of what you have and always, always smell good. She was Chanel No. 5. She worked, traveled, entertained, and loved. And her laugh was the most beautiful sound in the world. Her beauty transcends death.

LET THE SUN SHINE

We don't care how old she is this calendar year because Christie Brinkley remains the perfect California girl. What's her favorite beauty trick? Christie insists that one of her secret moves is to apply her makeup in bright sunlight. The natural light means you'll never slather on too much, aging yourself unnecessarily. Christie should know—even though she's in her 50s, she has the most natural, flawless look.

THE YOUNG AND THE GRAPEFRUIT

One of **Oprah Winfrey**'s favorite scents is Jo Malone's Grapefruit, and this may be the reason why:

A recent study at the Smell & Taste Treatment and Research Foundation in Chicago indicated: "When exposed to a whiff of pink grapefruit, the men in the study judged the women wearing it to be nearly six years younger than they actually were." So perfume can not only make you smell good, but it can make you look younger as well.

Overheard on the Red Carpet The socialites in New York are buzzing about their latest secret indulgence. It's fat injections, but not in the cheeks (face or rear end). They're getting the shots in their earlobes. The chic ladies who graze at Nobu say it's the first place their so-called friends check to see how old a woman really is. If she's got drooping lobes when she wears her 5-carat studs (and we don't mean her young, cute, male masseur) then she is definitely over 40 (God forbid). The Fifth Avenue girls now all head to their monthly appointments at the dermatologist to get injections in their ears. Price: $1,000. Having plumper earlobes to make your girlfriends believe you're younger . . . priceless.

MATERIAL GIRL HAIR

It's not easy being over 40 and still feeling like you're 24. Big stars, including **Madonna**, are fighting aging every step of the way. We all know about her intense yoga regime, but she also takes time out to make sure her tresses still look young, silky, and smooth by indulging in the Protein Hair Facial. It's a thirty-minute tress-transforming treatment offered at Privé Salons in New York City and Los Angeles. If you're there, give it a try—or ask your stylist about it.

OLD-SCHOOL BEAUTY

We love, love, love the Vermont Country Store catalog, and it's a favorite among celebrities.

Some of our favorite products sold in this amazing little tome include:

Tired Old Ass Soak

Talk about rejuvenation! This is a blend of salts that are chock-full of iron and trace minerals, plus 100 percent pure essential oils of rosemary and eucalyptus. Soak and you will feel like a new woman. You can also use it as a foot soak.

Sleeping Gloves

If your hands are dry and chapped, you can give yourself the glove. Smear the lotion on your hands, then pull on these cotton knit gloves and leave them on overnight. By morning your hands will feel silky smooth. This works in one treatment and the lotion won't rub off on your 500-thread-count sheets.

Bag Balm

Yes, we're talking cow udders. For years, farmers in Vermont have been rubbing Bag Balm on their mooing friends' udders to make them soft. You can use the same thing on rough, dry hands, elbows, knees, and feet.

Frownies and Wrinkies

Your mother probably used these years ago—just ask her! You can apply these Frownies to your forehead or between your eyes. Or try Wrinkies on the corners of your eyes and mouth. You just leave them on for a couple of hours or overnight and watch all those fine worry lines disappear before your eyes. They claim to work in three hours.

Overheard on the Red Carpet: She's an over-40 actress with the bod of a 20-year-old, but her under-eyes reveal her real age. To get rid of the telltale lines and bags under her eyes, her longtime makeup artist uses Angels Makeup Lifting Ampuls. They're the updated version of Frownies and help to instantly smooth wrinkles and firm and rehydrate the under-eye area. These ampuls are filled with secret ingredients like wheat germ protein and hydrogenated castor oil and collagen. You just soak the eye patches provided in the liquid and put them under your eyes for twenty minutes. Get these yourself (approximately $150) at www.angelsmakeup.com. **Rosario Dawson, Naomi Campbell, Elle MacPherson, Lucy Liu**, and **Kate Beckinsale** reportedly use these babies.

IMAGE MAKER: TAMMY BAKER NYE

A beauty pro for twenty years, Tammy Baker Nye has worked on countless celebrities for movies, TV, and concerts.

What are your five favorite products in your bathroom right now?

I use Cetaphil skin cleanser and baking soda and mix them together to form a paste. The baking soda acts as a mild exfoliant and the cleanser leaves my skin refreshed and clean.

If you had only $100 to spend on products, what would you buy first?

This is tough, but with much deliberation I would buy my Effexor. I have been a breast cancer survivor now for three years. I have to stay away from any type of hormone. My doctor prescribed for me Effexor and told me that this might help with hot flashes. I tried and low and behold it worked! Now the whole beauty process can begin without me being drenched!

What is the best antiaging tip you have?

The best antiaging advice I can give is don't smoke, wear sunscreen, and marry someone who is quick-witted and makes you laugh. Throw in a 9-year-old daughter and believe me, you won't feel a day over 29, maybe 31.

FRUGAL AND FABULOUS AFTER 40

We want you to have a lot of coin in your new Gucci purse. That's why we have these cost-saving tips tailored to help you put a few pennies away for tomorrow's beauty emergencies.

- What's in the bag? When it comes to a makeup bag, many Beverly Hills socialites and actresses spend big bucks on Prada, Chanel, and Marc Jacobs designer bags. But let's get down and dirty. Despite the chic names, after a short while, these makeup bags just get gunky and stained from the foundation, glosses, and accidentally opened blush tint. Here's a trick: Savvy girls go to the kids' department (of Target or Kmart) for school supplies and stock up on clear plastic see-through pencil cases. They're inexpensive, clean, and easy to toss and replace.

- To strengthen dry, peeling nails, soak your hands in warm milk and pat dry. If you're heading to the shower, hair conditioner is an amazing cuticle softener. Dab a little on in the shower and then push your cuticles back with a towel while drying off.

- Want to save a little money by extending the life of your pedicure? According to Carla Kay, a celebrity pedicurist in Los Angeles, you should wear insoles (Dr. Scholl's) all year long. They serve as a buffer between your foot and shoe and will help prevent calluses.

CELE-BEAUTY: CATHERINE HICKLAND

Millions of people the world over know Catherine Hickland from her work on the ABC daytime dramas *One Life to Live*, *Loving*, and *The City*, as well as countless guest appearances on other prime-time television series and movies of the week. She divides her time between New York and Los Angeles. (Did we mention she's also the proud mother of two dogs and five cats, all of whom she claims look like her?!)

A trained makeup artist and resident "Product Queen" at *Soap Opera Digest*, Cat recently realized a lifelong dream by launching her own custom-designed line of makeup and accessories, Cat Cosmetics. She recently released her makeover video, *Simply Gorgeous*, in retail stores nationwide.

What is a high-end, over-the-top expensive, just-can't-live-without purchase for beauty you've made, and why does it work so well for you?

I have been buying La Prairie Eye Cream for over ten years now, and at $125, it's considered high end. I believe in it. It's like this: You can spend $125 and have an eye cream that actually *does* something and lasts for six months or more, bringing the cost to 35 cents a day. I break it down because for most women $125 is a *lot* of money and sometimes you have to look at it like this. Even an average eye cream is going to cost at least $25 without the effectiveness. So bite the bullet. Save your sheckels and get the one that works . . . I love it because you can gently pat it over your makeup at the end of the day—a touch-up under the eye for a fresh look. It's miracle-working eye cream. End of story.

What is your favorite inexpensive or homemade beauty tip or product?

When I was making a movie in the Philippines, I noticed that Asian women had the most gorgeous, shiny hair that I have ever seen. Since the water there is so rough, I couldn't understand it, so I asked them. They put coconut oil in their hair, sometimes sleeping in it, or putting it in a ponytail for a few hours. We American chicks now have cold-pressed virgin coconut oil available to us in health-food stores for $6 to $10. It will last for twenty uses or more. You can cook with it, too. It's the healthiest oil in the world and great for people on diets. You can put it on your body as a moisturizer. What a bargain.

What does your beauty routine consist of on a daily and nightly basis?

My beauty routine starts with my mind, since I think that controls absolutely everything from the neck up and down. Aging is such a scary thing for most women, and actresses in particular, that I actually teach a workshop on how to reverse it by just using your mind. I always get up an hour before I need to and light a candle, meditate, and journal my thoughts. I get inside my gratitude and talk to God. That puts me in the world with my spiritual armor on, which basically makes me bulletproof to all the things that will come at me in a day. After meditating, I shower, moisturize my face and body, and put on whatever makeup I have time for that day. If I'm short on time, I always put on my glosses. They light up my face. Then I smoke up my eyes with Smolder, my smoky-eye-in-a-minute stick, and put on two coats of mascara. I brush on some bronzer and I'm out the door feeling like my bad self in two minutes. I always make sure I go to bed with a clean and moisturized face.

What are your all-time, top-five best beauty products that you can't live without?

La Prairie Eye Cream

Cat and Mouse Lip Gloss (Cat Cosmetics)

Girl on Fire Bronzer (Cat Cosmetics)

L'Oréal mascara

Smolder Smoky-eye-in-a-minute eye shadow stick (Cat Cosmetics)

If you were going to your own private island and could take only a limited beauty and skin-care "stash," what would you take with you?

CutieKit Custard Cream Body Butter (because my skin is so dry)

Vaseline Advanced Healing Body Lotion

All of the above-mentioned cosmetics

Mason Pearson hairbrush (boar bristles and nylon combo)

What is your secret antiaging tip?

Again, I adjust my mind first thing every morning. I'm not against plastic surgery, but I'm going to put it off as long as possible. And there are so many things we can do today without a scalpel. I love going to Renew Anti-Aging Salon in New York City for my microdermabrasion work. I also get the smallest amount of Botox injected into my forehead. But more important than anything, I keep my skin clean and moisturized.

What's your favorite health and diet tip?

Well, since I like to eat like a hog (think Arnold Ziffel) and all of my dishes are troughs, I have to stay on a diet plan that is actually a lifestyle. I have battled weight all of my life. I love Weight Watchers, but at twenty-one points it's not enough food for me. I get low blood sugar and need to eat five or six meals a day. The Zone Diet is good, but with my lifestyle, I can't stay faithful. Too much thinking. So the one that works for me is the Suzanne Somers Diet, which is food combining. It's easy, no real thinking required, and you get to eat . . . a lot! Her book, *Eat Great, Lose Weight*, is available in bookstores or at Amazon.com.

What do you do a month before, a week before, and the day of a big event to make sure you look your very best?

I hate working out. There, I said it. It bores me to tears. I will take one-on-one ballroom dancing lessons with a great choreographer and dance a few hours a day. That gets my arms really pretty, and my body, too. Dance is really a body transformer. A month before I may ramp up my diet routine and stick to it better to get a few pounds off. I like to wear showgirl dresses and they're kind of on the bare side. I make sure not to get a facial done too close to an event. It can often prompt a breakout or blotchiness, and I want to give it "settle-down" time. The day of the event, I make sure I have Bruce Wayne (my makeup artist) booked and just let him do his thing, using my cosmetics, of course. That's where I draw the line—literally! After he is finished, we put on the false eyelashes and I feel like a queen.

Tell us the biggest beauty blunder you see most women do on a daily basis.

Wearing purple- or blue-based lip color. Talk about aging yourself in one fell swoop! It duplicates the look of cardiac arrest. I find that women are really steeped in their lip-color habits. It's the hardest thing for me to get them to change when they come to me for a makeover. They are willing to give up everything but the lip color. It's like their blankie. Lightly lined lips and beautiful soft colors with a hint of frost in the center takes years off the face. Try it!

What is the craziest thing you've ever done for beauty?

I had collagen injected into my lips. Childbirth has to be more comfortable than having someone stick that needle in your lips. I looked like a platypus and it took two months to go away. I can always spot injected lips a mile away. They look like blowfish.

Give us the most unusual, unique, out-of-the-ordinary item you've ever used for beauty.

Desitin Ointment for baby diaper rash is awesome for dry cuticles.

HOLLYWOOD BEAUTY ICON: JANE RUSSELL

Jane Russell is one of the original Hollywood beauties. She dated Howard Hughes and shot movies with Marilyn Monroe and Howard Hawks. She paved the way for all the gorgeous women—or broads, as she calls them!—to follow in her high-heeled footsteps! Don't even get us started about her 18-hour bra.

In her 80s and living quietly in Santa Barbara, California, on her ranch, she is one of the ultimate beauty icons.

BB: So, Jane, you are a world-class beauty. What's your big secret?

Jane: (With a big hearty laugh and a long pause) Oh, honey. Sleep, lots of it, and hope your family has good genes!

BB: In the studio days, what were some of the great makeup secrets the artists used on you?

Jane: Well, I was 19 years old when I was doing movies, and the first day the makeup artist started working on me, it took him two hours. I wanted to get out of there a lot quicker, so I said thank you and started doing all my own makeup and I have ever since. I kept Shotgun [her makeup man], but basically he would get me my tea and yogurt for breakfast.

BB: What do you think about the styles and looks on the young starlets today?

Jane: Ridiculous! They have mud mouths. Dull, boring, flat-colored lipstick. They have hairdos that look like they just crawled out from under the bed, not on top of it. Those pointed high-heel shoes. They look like a bunch of witches. And the belly button rings! Oh, come on!

I never paid attention to style. I only used and did what was right for *me*!

BB: Jane, to this day you have a fabulous figure. Could you share a few of your diet tips with us?

Jane: I have never eaten much bread and I don't have a sweet tooth. I don't eat sugar. I will admit that my mother used to share a great piece of English toffee with me. But that was it for sweets.

BB: Howard Hughes designed a bra just for you. What do you think about the current Victoria's Secret styles?

Jane: Basically it's like the look I wore in *Outlaw* . . . the off-the-shoulder, loosely hanging . . . all the clothes had to look like they were falling off me. Because I had to wear all that kind of under-stuff for so long, now I wear clothing up to my neck and long sleeves.

BB: Tell us a secret you share only with your closet friends.

Jane: Married women should put their face on for their husbands when they are coming home from work. Remember, ladies, that they are around broads that have their faces on all day long. Put yours on, too!

BB: Okay, Jane give us one more.

Jane: This has nothing to do with a product or a cream. This has to do with your voice. The director **Howard Hawks** took all of us—**Lauren Bacall**, **Marilyn Monroe**, and myself—and said, "LOWER YOUR VOICE!" . . . **Lauren Bacall** still has the lowest voice of anyone I know to this day. The actresses of today all have these high-pitched baby-girl voices.

BB: What is your secret antiaging tip?

Jane: Wear color! The Lord made the mud and dirt brown and gray, then he made the flowers and the grass with lots of color. Take a lesson from him . . . wear color!

CHAPTER 7

Ready for Your Close-Up . . . Black Book Last-Minute Touch-Ups

Getting ahead in a difficult profession requires avid faith in yourself. You must be able to sustain yourself. Some people with mediocre talent, but with a great inner drive, go much further than people with vastly superior talent.

—**Sophia Loren**

I did think for a while that I should get boobs, but then I rejected the idea. It seemed like major surgery. But it's funny. When you talk about geting boobs with men they will say, "Oh, that's not a bad idea, but don't touch your face!

—**Julianne Moore**

We've covered skin, hair, and some extra tips if you've hit the big 4-Oh! Now, it's time to refine your program with a few *Black Book* red-carpet extras that will ensure that you take your good looks over the top.

A HOLLYWOOD BEAUTY MOMENT WITH HEIDI KLUM

BB: How do you decide what to wear for a big shindig?

Heidi: First, I keep an open mind. You never know how something will look until you put it on. I could say, "Oh that little black dress is boring. It's just another black cocktail dress." But then I put it on and the sleeves have a cut-out or part of the dress falls softly off my shoulders. Suddenly, I love this dress. So you have to take it on a case-by-case basis. Also, you don't have to go crazy with plaids and colors. Black can still be so great. Just a little holiday dressing tip, ladies!

BB: Do you ever feel a tad bit frumpy? Please say yes and we'll love you forever.

Heidi: Do I ever have an ugly day? Oh please! I'm wearing a hat today because I'm having a very bad hair day. There is just nothing I can do with it! But I try, because I know when I'm in public that it's my job. It's about creating a fantasy. But I'm like every other woman who sees flaws.

NAIL IT!

We like banana splits. We like doing splits. But when it comes to nail splits, we say *no mas*!

When your body's water content falls below 18 percent, nails become brittle, split, and peel. In autumn, there's a drop in humidity and the nail plate is prone to water loss.

The solution is to drink lots of water and apply a cream with alpha hydroxy acid to your nail bed every single day. Olive oil will do in a pinch.

BB Extra I: It's not hip to be square. You should always file your nails into an almond shape. It makes them look longer.

BB Extra II: Baking soda is a great nail scrub. The lightening agents take the yellow out of your nails in an instant. You can also get out an old toothbrush and rub whitening toothpaste on your finger- and toenails. It will whiten them immediately.

BROWBEATEN?

Eyebrow hair transplants are the hot new procedure in L.A. and Miami. There's an actual surgery to fill in sparse brows. Doctors take hair from the back of your head and implant it into your brow area. It takes about two hours and it's permanent. The cost is between $3,000 and $5,000 per pair (whew, not per brow).

THE RING THING

Does your favorite ruby cocktail ring slip and slide across your finger? Or are you afraid (banish the thought!) that the antique might actually fall off on the red carpet? Buy some Ring Guard Solution. It's a gel that you put inside the band of your ring. When you put the ring on it will stick to your finger, but it's easy to pull off. You can even use the stuff to keep ever-slipping earrings in place. Buy it for under ten bucks at www.earringsaccessories.com.

DESPERATE HOUSEWIVES' WINE

You want to look more beautiful and relaxed before a big event? Draw yourself a bath and pour some leftover red wine into the tub. The polyphenols found in grapes jump-start circulation to reveal healthier glowing softer skin. Pour one cup of red wine (don't worry about stains on skin or tub) into a warm bath, put a few rose petals on top, jump in, and stay in for twenty minutes. **Teri Hatcher** uses old wine and lets the sediments sink to the bottom of the tub. "I scoop them up in the tub and use them as an exfoliant. The only bad thing is you can't drink the whole bottle of wine," she tell us. But what price beauty?

BB Extra: You can also put rose petals in your bath to create the same effect as they do at famous spas in the Napa Valley.

GREEN ANTIAGE YOUR GENES

Bathe in cooled green tea. The antioxidants in the tea will stimulate your cells and rejuvenate them. The tannins in the tea tighten the skin and diminish wrinkles. (Could we pour it all over our faces? Just kidding.) Steep five or six green tea bags in a warm bath, soak for twenty minutes, and add anti-aging boosters by putting a few orange slices in the tea for a vitamin C boost.

CRAMPS, REVAMPED

Want to ease mind-numbing cramps? We can't alleviate your worries about wearing white, your endless need for chocolate, or the zits on your face at age 36 (isn't being a woman grand?), but we can offer a suggestion that Hollywood stars know about combating the cramps and hormonal surges. A New York aromatherapist and shiatsu therapist gave us Girl Balm, which she swears takes away some of the pain. Massage a gob of it on your lower belly. It's made out of hemp seed oil, jojoba, unrefined beeswax, and the essential oils of clarity sage, rose geranium, gingerroot, and black pepper. The idea is to re-create balance for your ever-active hormones and help with circulation to get rid of any icky feelings, aches, and perhaps even the need to toss a coffee cup at your husband (although we can only make so many promises). Perhaps it can put a period on your . . . period. You can order it online at www.buddhanose.com.

LOSING YOUR MARBLES IN A GOOD WAY

Manis and pedis and facials. How can we even afford to pay the mortgage? And there comes a time when a girl just can't find enough time to schedule in all her beauty appointments because you still have to eat and watch reruns of *Sex and the City.*

If you must skip your tootsie treatment, you can give yourself a relaxing pedicure at home with some simple childhood toys.

Yes, go out and buy a bag of marbles! Fill a little basin with warm water and some oils. Add the marbles, then dip your toes in. Slide your feet over the marbles, which will create the same physical reaction as a wonderful pedicure at Beauty Bungalow, where **Rachel Griffiths** and **Sarah Wynter** get the famous Spa Pedicure. The marbles, just like any good pedicure, will hit the pressure points on your feet. Once these points are massaged by human hands or marbles, your entire body will calm down and relax.

IMAGE MAKER: CHERYL WOODCOCK

From her beach house in Mexico, we present *Entertainment Tonight* and *The Insider* producer-extraordinaire **Cheryl Woodcock**:

"My name is **Cheryl Woodcock**. I live in Beverly Hills, California, and work on the beautiful and historical Paramount lot. I have produced *Entertainment Tonight* (the number one syndicated entertainment news program worldwide) for the last seven years. I also produce *The Insider*. I'm also one of the correspondents for both shows. As you can see, I have my hands full, producing, directing, writing, getting hair and makeup every single day; keeping myself in tip-top shape for the camera, red carpets, junkets, interviews; keeping my celebrities happy; keeping my executive producers happy; charity events; social lunches; running two households with staff, carpool, and, first and foremost, taking care of my family. I'm a mother first! I'm incredibly happily married to a man who spent the last thirty-eight years in the TV business. We also have a fabulous beach house in Punta Mita, Mexico, near the Four Seasons, where we run every chance we get—end of sweeps, spring break, etc."

What is a high-end, over-the-top expensive, just-can't-live-without purchase for beauty you've made and why does it work so well for you?

RéVive skin-care line—the entire regime. It is very expensive—around $3,000 every few months. The Intensité face and eye creams are dreamy. These products keep my skin looking radiant. The fabulous Dr. Greg Brown designed the line to keep women my age nearing 40 away from the knives and needles, although a little hyloform/collagen here and there is not a bad thing right before the Oscars or Golden Globes.

What is your favorite inexpensive or homemade beauty tip or product?

Aquaphor and plain old Vaseline. I learned about Aquaphor from my celebrity peditrician, Dr. Peter Waldstien. I use it all over my children for dryness, healing, and a whole host of issues. Every single day, after I bathe, I smother my feet on top and on the bottom with Aquaphor. Then I put on my Havaianas [plastic flip-flops] and get myself ready. This keeps my feet looking fabulous and moist for those beautiful Manolo Blahniks that will soon be placed upon my feet. I use Vaseline every single night on my nails and cuticles to keep my hands looking young. I also like to use virgin olive oil on my face every night for a week leading up to a red-carpet event. It keeps your face looking young and vibrant.

What does you beauty routine consist of on a daily and nightly basis?

My beauty regime in the A.M. consists of RéVive skin care, one emergency packet, vitamins, and a healthy breakfast. I do the same thing at night—adding Vaseline on the hands. Once a week I use a mud body mask all over my face and entire body. This takes about twenty minutes. Caution—keep hubby and children out of the bathroom as it's quite a frightful sight. I look like a Zulu woman being sacrificed.

What are your all-time, never-fail, top-five best beauty products that you can't live without?

RéVive skin care, YSL concealer, MAC Belightful Iridescent Powder, Chanel foundation, NARS Orgasm blush, Aquaphor.

What is your secret antiaging tip?

My secret antiaging product is virgin olive oil and Vaseline, Aquaphor, RéVive Intensité.

What sets a socialite, or a true beauty who all the other girls look at, apart from the pack?
Style and NO FEAR.

Tell us about the biggest beauty blunder you think women make.
The biggest beauty blunder that women do is too much makeup and too many stylists! Too many cooks in the kitchen. Keep it simple before the big event.

What is the craziest thing you've ever done for beauty?
The craziest thing I have ever done for beauty was a colonic before the Oscars this year. It was just awful and very painful. The woman who was directing the procedure was so mean and kept telling me to keep my mouth shut and stop telling her about my bodily functions. I was lying there and just thought this was the lowest of the low for beauty. I would not recommend this procedure to anyone ever again! I tried Botox once . . . I was so worried that I would get sick from it.

Finish this sentence: I feel red-carpet ready when . . .
I feel red-carpet ready when the Harry Winston jewels have arrived, my stylist Anya Berger has approved everything, Pam Farmer—my favorite makeup artist—is packing up, and the car has arrived at the gate. I also know that I have been very diligent over the past week and all my hard work has paid off. I'm usually very hungry.

What is your favorite at-home, in-a-quick-pinch home remedy for beautiful skin or hair?

Home remedy for hair is to do a protein pack twice a week. I put the cream on my hair and sleep in it. Virgin olive oil for the face. I forgot to say that I pray every morning. I say a prayer before I walk into the studio and I say a prayer before I walk the red carpet or before I interview anyone. Prayer and meditation keep me centered.

What is the craziest product you've ever used for beauty?
The craziest thing is Preparation H under my eyes. It really takes the swelling down for those early-morning call times.

SLEEP WITH US—PART ONE

Sleeping Beauty was onto something. You need your rest in order to jump-start your beauty routine. What can you do while you slumber? Start snoring and follow along.

FEET: You can put lotion on your feet and then snuggle them into a thick pair of socks to make sure the product sinks deeply into your tootsies.

HANDS: Rub some shea butter or great hand cream on your hands and nails before you go to sleep. You can slip some beauty gloves on to make sure the lotion sinks in while you get your REM sleep. If you want to skip the gloves, put on the lotion a few minutes before getting into bed so you won't mess up your sheets.

ZITS: Put on some acne lotion with salicylic acid before you go to sleep. You might even wake up in the morning with the eruption gone.

NECK: Find thick, creamy face lotion and rub it on your neck before you go to sleep. It's one of the first places that women age, so it's better to do this sooner rather than later.

HAIR: Get a deep-conditioning hair product, olive oil, or Neem oil and massage into your scalp.

BB Extra: Protect your Calvin Klein pillowcases by wrapping up your hair in an old scarf. Don't use the designer Pucci one!

NAILS: Put some specialty nail oil, olive oil, Neem oil, or coconut oil on your nail bed to make them stronger and nourish them while you get your z's.

LIPS: Follow the lead of **Tyra Banks** or **Calista Flockhart**. Dab some good old-fashioned Vaseline on your kisser. Or try the more expensive overnight treatments for lips, to soften and exfoliate.

LET ME SLEEP

Okay, everyone from **Catherine Zeta-Jones** to **Jennifer Lopez** has told us that sleep is their number-one beauty secret. But how are you supposed to be a sleeping beauty when you have kids, a dog, a job, and a husband? Did we mention the dog?

Here's a trick: Instead of popping a sleeping pill that leaves you groggy and can be addictive, drink half a glass of water, put a pinch of salt on your tongue, and let it dissolve. Make sure the granules don't press against the roof of your mouth.

Studies have shown that the combination of water and salt alters the electrical charge of the brain, inducing a deep slumber.

Zzzzzzzzzzzzz.

SLEEP WITH US—PART TWO

According to the National Sleep Foundation, 74 percent of Americans have trouble sleeping. We have a few special secrets . . .

Mix a drop of lavender essential oil with water in a spray bottle and spray your pillowcase from a distance. When you lie down the scent will tell your brain to relax. Zzzzzzzz.

From Vanessa Getty to Faye Dunaway, some of the most beautiful women in the world say that sleeping on your back is one of the best ways to combat wrinkles and creases in the face. If you sleep facedown smashed into the pillow, then invest in a satin pillowcase. Your face will slide on the case, thus discouraging wrinkles.

Putting a drop or two of eucalyptus oil on your pillow will help to clear stuffy nasal passages if you have the flu or allergies. Scientists say that when you have a cold, you can wake up as many as a hundred times a night without knowing it. The eucalyptus will help you breathe clearly all night long.

BB Extra: In the morning, if you have bloodshot lids, apply a tea bag of raspberry tea that has been put in the freezer. The red will be gone in a few minutes.

CELE-BEAUTY: TRACEY BREGMAN

With her signature long red spiral locks, our friend and Emmy winner Tracey Bregman plays a department store heiress named Lauren Fenmore and jumps from hot soaps *The Young and the Restless* to *The Bold and the Beautiful* with the greatest of ease. She can also be found at her Malibu mansion where her best role is as the mother of two young sons. Tracey always looks gorgeous and doesn't mind sharing why.

What are your five favorite products in your bathroom right now?
The Leaf & Rusher skin-care line, Dr. Harold Lancer skin products. I'm like a mad scientist in my bathroom every night. Beach sunless tan, Nutura Bissé body cream. Believe me, there's a lot more than five but I love them all.

If you had only $100 to spend on products, what would you buy first?
First, I'd cry. I'm so high maintenance that I need a gold bullion to pay for my products. If push came to shove, it would be under-eye cream and sunblock.

What is the best antiaging tip you have?
Sunblock, sunblock, and sunblock! Did I say sunblock?!
And I use a hydrating under-eye cream.

Please tell us one secret beauty tip that you share with only your closest friends.
I buy Na-PCA spray from Whole Foods. My husband uses it on his face after he shaves and I use it on my bikini area. Keeps me baby smooth and no ingrowns or rough skin.

CHAPTER 8

How to Have a Baby
and Stay an A-List Babe

You're either sexy or you're a mother. I don't want to have to choose, so I challenged that theory.

—**Demi Moore**, a woman we love

If I get to take a shower, it's a big deal. Just ask any mother of young children.

—**Felicity Huffman**

RUNNING HOT AND COLD

It's funny that sometimes the hottest women on the planet get icy cold when it comes to their beauty tips. **Kate Hudson** insists that when her son, Ryder, keeps her awake all night teething before a shoot the next morning, her first line of defense isn't to swim into a jar of expensive cream to get rid of her puffy eyes and skin. "It sounds completely old fashioned, but my mom told me this one years ago and it works," **Hudson** tells us. "You just get out a bowl and fill it with ice. Wash your face with the ice water and—poof—the puff is gone." (Since her mother is legendary beauty **Goldie Hawn**, we bow to her as a beauty goddess and have our ice makers working 24-7. We can barely even fit anything else into our freezers.) **Kate** might also entertain an advanced trick from a Los Angeles makeup artist. If your face feels really puffy, hold an ice cube against the roof of your mouth with your tongue. The chill actually helps reduce the swelling from the inside out, and the effect will last all day long.

BOUNCING ALONG

When you have a baby, you're constantly doing laundry. The product Bounce softens and adds a great smell to your little one's teeny clothes, but it's also a great way to smooth static electricity in your hair. Swipe a Bounce sheet down your hair shaft and the flyaways are gone, gone, gone. (You can also put this into sneakers that are getting a workout from all that stroller rolling to make them smell great the next day.)

BB Extra: How do those new Hollywood mommies get so skinny, so fast? Well, we needed to know, too, so we put on our undercover Burberry trench coats and headed into the Beverly Hills manicured trenches to find out. It turns out that celebrity moms order Bohemian Baby, the must-have home-delivered baby food of Hollywood's A-listers. It's organic, tasty, and has hardly any calories. It's already portion-controlled so the mommies are asking for double deliveries: one for the future president of Sony and one for mommy. With choices like pomegranate-pear puree and cuban black beans with green veggies and coconut korma, moms are wolfing the tykes' tasty treats and that's all they're eating till they reach their goal weight. (Hollywood Beauty Speak: Dropping the Baby Weight.

Never go out in public weighing over 112 pounds even after giving birth. It's a major unspoken rule!)

CINDY'S SPRITZ

Supermodel **Cindy Crawford** has the most beautiful skin that's always fresh and dewy, even after having two babies. One of her secrets is a small, purse-size spray bottle filled with leftover milk from her kid's bottles and equal part mineral water. She sprays it over her face and neck during the day. It adds moisture and plumpness to her already gorgeous skin.

STRETCHING IT

When you're married to **The Donald**, the only thing that needs stretching is the bottom line. That's why **Mrs. T**, **Melania**, who recently gave birth to a baby Barron, slathered her pregnant midsection with a product called Belly Butter. Made from pure essential oils of lavender, sweet orange, and mandarin, the product is a celeb's dream before and after childbirth. (By the way, it works on all skin that has expanded and contracted, so it's great to use during weight loss, too.) It promises no stretch marks, and smart mamas know to use it before and after giving birth. And we love the name of the company that makes this got-to-get-it goo—Bella Mama. Other products from the woman-owned company include Nursing Salve, Belly Oil, Foot Salts, and one of our favorite new-mama gift packages, the Just Hatched! Gift Set.

TEETHING RINGS

Baby is teething and you're getting no sleep at all. When baby is done, put the teething rings back in the freezer, and use them on your own eyes to reduce swelling and puffiness. You might still be doing this when your child is 18 and you're waiting up for him all night.

NUMB AND NUMB-ER

You used to have beautifully coiffed brows, but weeks after giving birth there has been no time to go see Damon Roberts in Beverly Hills for a quick brow job. Now you have a forest growing up there and you don't know where to start. You get out the tweezers and . . . ouch! What to do, what to do? Dab a little Anbesol on the brow and pluck away pain free. Hey, haven't you suffered enough with childbirth?

SAVING GRACE

Kym's friend **Elisabeth Hasselbeck** from *The View* and of *Survivor* fame has a gorgeous baby daughter named Grace. She uses Aquaphor to stay dewy. It's a rich cream that protects baby's skin from the wind, cold, and sun. Moms love it as a lip smoother, and you can also put it under your eyes for a blast of moisture. It's also perfect for chapped hands.

LICK YOUR PROBLEMS

Your young child probably loves popsicles, but there's a way Mom can use them, too, for beauty. If you're stressed out, grab one and suck on it. The tension from the sucking will cause your jaw muscles to stiffen and constrict the vessels that supply oxygen to your brain. The cold from the popsicle then causes stiff tissues to relax. This sequence will improve your circulation and calm you. Until the next temper tantrum.

OH BABY, SHAMPOO

Your baby has beautiful blond hair like you used to when you had time to go to the salon for a touch-up. Now you're doing those roots yourself and your hair has turned orangey or brassy. If you've messed up your color, then simply suds up with baby shampoo. Wash your hair several times with it and your hair will readjust its pH balance.

BB Extra: Baby shampoo is also strong but gentle enough to wash out your delicate lingerie and makeup brushes.

BRUSH YOUR CARES AWAY

So you're not feeling like sexy **Pam Anderson** after giving birth. Well, Pam can still serve as your role model in the Mom department. Pam told us how busy moms can have sexy hair in a flash. Grab one of your child's old baby toothbrushes, spray some hair spray onto the bristles, and then take a section of the hair at the crown of your head and tease. The bristles are so small and gentle that they allow the teasing to take place at the roots, adding subtle height and volume. No word on how you'll look in the red *Baywatch* suit.

BB Extra: Baby toothbrushes are great for cleaning jewelry. Remember to throw out the toothbrush when you're done.

OIL CHANGE

Take the baby oil from your baby's bath and use it on a cotton ball as eye-makeup remover. It gets rid of even the toughest mascara and heaviest eye makeup without drying out the delicate skin around the eye.

DIAPER DUTY

Picking up and putting down baby can hurt your back and make it ache. Don't even get us started on your aching shoulders and neck. Instead of grabbing the heating pad, take a cotton baby diaper, wet it a bit and put it in the microwave for thirty seconds. Then apply the diaper to your aching area.

BB Extra: By the way, this is also good for cramps. Lay it right on your tummy.

Overheard on the Red Carpet: What 1970s beauty angel and mother of many young 'uns still looks fabulous in her later ages without too much knife work on her famous face? Insiders say that the lack of crow's-feet and expression lines across her magnificent mug aren't due to Botox or cosmetic enhancements either. This beauty swears by not allowing any expressions to cross her face. She's so bland in her facial movements that she looks like a pristine statue. We think we'll go for more of exuberant personality even if it gives us a few extra fine lines.

CHAPTER 9

What Would Sarah Jessica Parker Do?

I cried every morning before school. I could never find my shoes, my socks, my hair ribbons, my homework . . . and my sister always saved me.

—**SJP,** our style hero

Every single day we're faced with excruciating beauty situations. What should we wear? How should we accessorize? How much is too much (fill in the blank)?

When it's almost too much to cope with, we simply stand in our favorite room of the house (the bathroom) and the dilemma is solved by saying these magic words: What would Sarah Jessica Parker do? (We do this sober and without a cosmo nearby.)

It's no secret that Carrie, uh, we mean Sarah, has been our style icon for years. She gave us the flower, the name necklace, the good-luck horseshoe necklace, Manolos for day wear, and even horizontal stripes—worn to perfection when she got off the plane in Paris with perfect makeup and non-frizzed tumbling curls.

Sarah, we're humbled by you and we want to live our

lives the SJP way. We would kiss your feet, but why ruin a good pair of $450 shoes?

This chapter is devoted to mind-boggling beauty dilemmas, and we've asked the experts to help us imagine what Sarah might do. We even got a few tips from SJP herself.

So stylish. So nice. What more can we say? Except, can we borrow those silver Manolos with the little circle thing in the front that were made especially for you for the Tatum O'Neal episode of *Sex and the City*? Sorry, but we had to ask.

EXPIRATION, DATE

One of the toughest beauty challenges you face on a date is the kissing vs. lipstick dilemma. You want to look nice and wear lipstick, but you don't want to leave it all over your date if you give him a kiss hello or good-bye.

What to do? Jeanine Canter, top Hollywood makeup artist, says ladies shouldn't give too much lip service while preparing for a big date. Forget the sticky, shiny, shimmering gloss that men rate as a huge turn-off—they don't want to get it all over their faces. Instead, she advises to use a little bit of lip liner all over your lip with a sheer gloss over it. That way your guy won't feel like he's jumping into a mouthful of goopy makeup. We're sure Aidan would approve.

SMELLING SWEET

When asked where a woman should wear perfume, Coco Chanel quickly had the best reply. She said, "Wherever she wants to be kissed." It's good advice to please the Mr. Big in your life.

THE GREAT KATE (SHE'S NOT SJP! BUT WE STILL LOVE HER)

Kate Beckinsale, so perfect that she should insure her entire being, says that two or three baths a day make her a very stress-free English lass. Her serenity even prevents beauty disasters. Kate tells us her bath is either filled with Epsom salts, Jo Malone grapefruit oil (see, we were right about Jo), or Moroccan Rose Otto bath oil by Ren. Out of the bath, her director hubby has a yen for **Jessica Simpson,** but it's not what you think. He likes when **Kate** uses **Jessica's** Dessert line of body scents. "He will literally come at me with a fork when I wear the one that smells like cake batter," **Kate** says.

GUCCI, CALVIN, AND GALLIANO (WHEN YOU'RE NOT A STICK FIGURE)

Patricia Field was the hot stylist for *Sex and the City* and put all that Chanel, Galliano, and Christian Louboutin on **Anne Hathaway** for the movie *The Devil Wears Prada.* Patricia says girls with curvy figures like **Anne** should "go for clothing with a defined waistline and fabrics that are soft or well tailored." Another hint for eveningwear: "A deeper V also accentuates curves in a great way," says Patricia.

EXTRA PADDING

You think your Stayfree mini pad just wants to sit around in your $150 pair of La Perla underwear? *No, sisters.* Those pads want to be free for other uses. If your underarms sweat a lot, attach a pad inside the armpit of your clothing. The mini pad will absorb perspiration and stop you from staining the expensive material. For a red-carpet event, wear a satin nude-colored pad in the arms of your dress. It's small, will stick easily, and prevents sweat stains.

BB Extra: Put a mini pad in your Manolos or other high heels or boots. They'll absorb odor, stop your tootsies from hurting, and even add a little bit to your height.

HANDS ACROSS AMERICA

Ever notice that in the middle of winter your hands are so tough that it feels like you've been working the land for the last month—with no gloves? Never fear because your morning habit will help get rid of this condition. Yes, brew yourself a hot cup of java in the A.M. and then place the cooled grounds in a plastic bag, which you'll stick in the fridge. Two times a week, scoop out a teaspoon of your used coffee grounds, which you'll rub around your hands. Think of it as a hand exfoliator! When you're done, just run your hands under some cool water for a few seconds and marvel at how the tannic acid in the coffee has removed the dead cells from your mitts.

SARAH SITUATIONS SOLVED!

Sarah Jessica Parker recently told Cindy that there are two things you never do after a certain age. Start with shorty-short skirts. "At a certain age, a really short skirt doesn't serve you very well," SJP says.

And then there is the matter of a certain colored cell phone, which, incidentally, Sarah's character, Carrie Bradshaw, did carry in an episode of *Sex and the City*.

"If I carried a pink cell phone, that'd be crazy," Sarah opines. "That's for Lindsay Lohan. She's the age. And she should carry a pink cell phone."

It doesn't serve you well after you're out of your Lindsay years. Got it?

When you grow up and you're different, all you want to do is find a way to be the same. And then as a more mature adult, you realize the beauty of thinking on your own.

—**SJP**, our red-carpet role model

SNAGGED IGNITION

You're in the limo on your way to the Burgundy Room (Hollywood Beauty Speak: Weeknight engagement; i.e., if it is a Tuesday night, you have to be going to the Burgundy Room. It's the only night to go there.) and God forbid, but you have a chipped nail and of course the limo driver is unprepared. No diamond nail file to be found. Grab yourself a book of matches on your way into the club. The ignition strip is slightly abrasive, so it will smooth any rough edges. Now, the only rough edge in your life will be that catty girl across the bar checking out your guy.

STRESS 'N' SMELL

Stressed out and have to look gorgeous for the evening with your version of Mr. Big, or even Mr. Medium? Sniff a dryer sheet and watch your stress level drop by 19 percent. Strange, but true: A study at Chicago's Smell & Taste Treatment and Research Foundation discovered that many people associate the dryer sheet smell with home. It may prompt happy memories that produce soothing brain waves and make you feel calmer. Or let it rip. Tear a few dryer sheets into long strips. Don't think about anything and you'll feel calmer in minutes from the combo of ripping and smelling.

UNDER PROTECTION

Nobody wants to smell bad, but it's a bit unsettling to read reports that allegedly link underarm deodorants and antiperspirants with breast cancer. Now, many women are racing to their local health-food stores and Trader Joe's to switch to all-natural or organic underarm protection. Crystal natural stones, nonaerosol sprays, and even all-natural solid gels are becoming more popular. Many women feel it's better to be safe than sorry.

BRUSH YOUR BOD

You're feeling a little sluggish and have a special event to attend, but you're just not running around singing "I Feel Pretty." There is an all-natural way to improve your looks and your flow of energy. Dry-brush your body before you step into the shower in the morning. With a long-handled natural bristle brush or loofah, brush your legs, then arms, from the tips of your fingers and toes toward the heart. Brush your torso toward the heart. Be gentle with the breast area and avoid the face. Your body will tingle slightly from your revved-up circulation and you'll have your own inner glow!

THE MILE-HIGH BEAUTY CLUB

Helen Jeffries, makeup artist to Hollywood's elite, including Matt LeBlanc, Jet Li, and Governor Ah-nuld Schwarzenegger, knows that the friendly skies aren't so friendly to your skin. What to do if you're jet-setting from coast to coast? Helen advises, "I always take an eye cream and a good moisturizer in my bag. I'll also pack MAC cleansing wipes and Clear Face. Every few hours, I focus on my face and clean it with the wipes and then moisturize. The bottom line is your face gets filthy on planes because there is so much of the jet fuel in the air and it settles into your skin. The recycled air is also so drying to your skin."

Helen also brings a spray bottle of Evian to moisturize her face. "I've also created my own little spritzer bottles filled with mineral water and a little bit of oil. That's a great thing to spray on your skin during a long flight." She adds a good eye cream to the mix because the skin under your peepers tends to get very puffy at 35,000 feet.

Helen says that really getting rid of that pasty airplane look should happen once you safely reach your five-diamond hotel suite or the local Holiday Inn Express. "The first thing I do when I get to the hotel after an airplane ride is to exfoliate my face. Get out the scrub and get all of that airplane and airport grime out of your pores and then moisturize. You will instantly look prettier and lose most of that jet-lag look."

NOT SO SURE

You're wearing your favorite black John Galliano cocktail dress and before you leave the house, you decide to go for one last teeny swipe of deodorant. Suddenly, you have a white streak near your armpit that's slid onto the outside and inside of your frock. Deep breath. Don't panic. Just grab a baby wipe, which has just enough non-color-fading, non-material-destroying juice in it to get rid of the stain without hurting the material.

MORE WITH SARAH!

So many questions for **SJP**, so little time.

BB: What has been your biggest beauty disaster?

SJP: Once, I ran down the block in these heels and woke up in the middle of the night in agony. I had torn the tendons in my foot. It was a little reminder that I'm not 27. I'm 40. But I'll never stop wearing heels.

BB: What do you carry in your purse?

SJP: I always have a tissue, a pacifier, and a lip gloss, and some Orbit gum in case I have bad breath.

POOR BUT HAPPY

Are you getting stress lines worrying about money? Consider this fact: Individuals usually get richer during their lifetimes, but not happier. According to a study from the *British Medical Journal*, which studied people in forty-four countries, family life was the greatest source of satisfaction in people's lives, not moola. So it proves that family and friends are better for your health than money!

CELE-BEAUTY: DAISY FUENTES

Model, spokesperson, and clothing, fragrance, and jewelry designer **Daisy Fuentes**, whose line is sold at Kohl's, has always been a role model in our beauty eyes. In the midst of her doing ten million different things, she graciously stopped in her Jimmy Choos to answer a few questions about how she always looks flawlessly gorgeous.

What are your five favorite products in your bathroom right now?
Natura Bissé body cream
Crème de la Mer facial moisturizer
Crème de la Mer tinted sunscreen for the face with SPF 18
Queen Helene Mint Julep Masque
Kiehl's Cream with Silk Groom

If you had only $100 to spend on products, what would you buy first?
Moisturizer for the face and body. Some less-expensive drugstore brands are very good like Olay with 30 SPF and Nivea Q10 body-firming lotion. Shu Uemura mascara; Neutrogena Moisturizing Lip Gloss; bronzer.

What is your best antiaging tip?
SPF—at least 20. I *always* put it on my face and chest. No drugs and alcohol. Lots of water and plenty of sleep. Love and happiness definitely help.

Tell us about your biggest beauty blunder.
I used baby oil for suntan lotion. Yes, even on my face! And I got a perm on my naturally super-curly hair, plus long acrylic nails. I could go on and on.

What is the most unusual item you've ever used on yourself or someone else to make them look more beautiful?
I've heard that some of the contestants on Miss Universe use Preparation H under their eyes for puffiness . . . weird! I haven't tried it myself and I really can't imagine how puffy my eyes would have to get for me to even consider it.

Have you ever had a 911 beauty emergency?
Never had any! Knock on wood!

SMELLY NELLY

For those of us who unfortunately dive into the bottle of perfume by mistake, there is a solution that doesn't include hiding out alone in the house with even your pets shunning you for days. Instead rub some unscented body lotion over the skin where you over-sprayed the scent. The lotion will neutralize the smell, but not to the point where your perfume will go away. In other words, you don't need to do a re-spray before you leave the house or you'll be back where you started in Smell Town.

And here's another quick fix if you've tipped the bottle a little bit too much. Just grab a lemon. The juice is acidic and helps cut the fragrance's oil. Wash with soap and water, then take off what's left with a lemon juice–soaked cotton ball.

AND A FINAL WORD FROM SJP ON HER FASHION GURU

"My son, James Wilke, will take one look at me in the morning and say, 'Take that dress off. I just don't like it. I want you to wear down pants today.' Down pants means long pants. He doesn't want to see any skin. He will say, 'Mommy, I see part of your belly.'

"My son is also obsessed with the Beatles, so he thinks he should only dress like a Beatle. He wants all of us to dress like Beatles. We're talking the *Yellow Submarine* era, which is big collars with flowers on them. Wait, I already did flowers on *Sex and the City*!"

CHAPTER 10

The Black Book of Hollywood Diet Secrets

What's the best cure for cellulite? Pants.
> **—Meredith Vieira** of *The Today Show*

Don't be ashamed if you're a little thick. I like the thickness, too. Just a little girth is what I need, something to keep me warm in the winter. I like legs and dumps. Dumps is like the posterior. I would say "derriere" for you.
> **—Jamie Foxx**

Dessert? I eat three M&M's a day.
> **—Denise Richards**

I'm all about fashion, cheeseburgers, and bright red lipstick.
> **—Scarlett Johansson**

We're not trying to be a diet book, but during the course of culling the world's best beauty tips, the celebs and their people couldn't wait to divulge their most amazing diet secrets to us. What could we do except write them down and share them with you?

We collected these weight-loss tips over the course of a year, and what follows are the best of the best. By the way, we're currently in the process of writing down the thousand other body and diet secrets the stars told us for a follow-up book. Until then, here's a taste to get you started.

HOLD THE OIL, PASS THE VINEGAR

So you're at your favorite restaurant or about to go to a big party and you're worried about pigging out on all the high-fat, high-carb foods. If possible, start with a salad covered with a vinegar-based of dressing. This will cut your appetite because the acid in vinegar keeps your blood sugar level for two hours, says the *European Journal of Clinical Nutrition*. Don't pass the cheese puffs! If you don't think the vinegar dressing will be available at your event, have a salad with this dressing before you leave the house.

JUMP IT OFF

If you're about to go on a big date, to a wedding or to a family reunion, try this little Hollywood trick to guarantee you'll look your most fabulous best: Jump on a mini trampoline for about fifteen minutes a few mornings before the big soiree. It's a great way to get exercise and it's said to reduce bloating and water retention quickly and naturally. The mini tramp's approximate cost is $39. Flat belly at the big date or family reunion . . . priceless!

AN APPLE CIDER A DAY

Soap star **Michelle Stafford** of *The Young and the Restless*, who has a killer bod, insists that many mornings she drinks eight ounces of hot water mixed with a tablespoon of apple cider vinegar and the juice from half of a lemon. "It reduces the toxins from my glands and gives me so much energy," she says. "It also helps me lose weight."

BANK ON IT

Tyra Banks crowns *America's Next Top Model*, so who better to pass on a few tips about looking your best? To get rid of cellulite on the butt or thighs, she has made a scrub out of coffee grounds. The chemicals pull the toxins out of the body and the fine grounds help stimulate circulation and minimize the appearance of bumpy, cottage cheese–like textures that come with age.

BB Extra: Coffee has been said to fend off certain types of skin cancers, too.

GETTING YOUR Z

Hmmm, we always wondered how one week a celebrity looked a little normal (Hollywood Beauty Speak: Chunky) and then just a week and a half later, the same celebrity, model, or wannabe shows up at a big, high-exposure event looking thin, trim and flat-tummied. Well, we found out one of Hollywood's dirty little secrets. The hottest, trendiest, sure-fire way to lose those unwanted extra pounds is a *sore throat*! We don't mean a real sore throat, but a fake one, silly.

The starlets save their real Academy Award–winning per-formances for when they call the doctor and have to act like they have the worst sore throat and are in desperate and im-mediate need of medication—not just any medication, but a Z-Pak. Everyone worth their water weight knows that a pre-scription for the antibiotic Zithromax, which is a five-day course designed to rid the body of harmful bacteria, also im-mediately cuts your appetite, eliminates cravings, and takes your hunger away completely. *You just don't want to eat.*

Not that we're docs, but we hear the desire for food can sometimes stay away for a week after you've stopped the med-ication. One up-and-coming pin-thin starlet confesses, "I do it about four times a year for the quick fix. I mean I have to fit into the new, skin-tight Versace and nothing can help me ex-cept my 'Z.'" A Beverly Hills doctors who dispenses the stuff says, "I can't believe the Hollywood elite would endure nau-sea, stomach cramps, and frequent trips to the bathroom let alone knowing that too much use of the antibiotic renders it ineffective and leaves them vulnerable to infections." Then he pauses and says, "Actually, it's Hollywood. I can imagine it."

SALMON-ELLA

We've found surprising evidence that models don't just live on mints, cigarettes, and coffee. No, it's not Diet Coke. Time to spill the low-carb, fat free, totally organic beans. A British model tells us she just carries tins of fish with her. She admits the fish food isn't great for her breath, but the super-skinny size 000 doesn't care. She says, "I carry my salmon or mackerel and it stops me from snacking on high-calorie fattening foods. It's great for your skin and hair." So there.

GIVE US A C

Here is a trick that TV actresses know works because the camera really does add an extra ten pounds to your frame. Top trainers in Hollywood will tell their clients, including A-list young actresses, to put down their cans of diet soda. Instead, mix into a liter of Evian or sparkling water exactly two packets of a vitamin powder called Emergen-C. (It's available nationwide at Trader Joe's and other drugstores.) One TV personality we know dropped a quick fifteen pounds in just four weeks by drinking this! Of course, she also ate sensibly and hit the gym a few times. But the C also worked wonders on her. At Arizona State University, a study revealed that only 500 mgs of vitamin C (which is only half the packet of Emergen-C) burned fat one-third faster and that subjects using this tool were even more motivated to exercise! Excuse us now while we race to the store.

BB Extra: Everyone should ditch the diet soda. It not only bloats you, but certain studies show that the artificial sweeteners make you hungrier and reduce the release of fat in your body.

J.LOW DOWN

We all know that J.Lo has great discipline and works out regularly with various trainers. One of her favorites is celebrity trainer Gunnar Peterson. She is so committed to staying lean that even when she is shooting a movie, she sets up her training sessions with Gunnar at his Beverly Hills state-of-the-art private gym, as early as 4:30 A.M . . . That's before she puts in a whole day on the set. Talk about commitment and discipline. (So next time you moan about getting up early to go to the gym just think about J.Lo.) Another little insider tip is that when J.Lo is trying to drop a few pounds, she gets on a strict three-day regimen of eating eight mini meals a day with no cheating. The meals often consist of cereal, omelets, and hot skim milk.

EAT, EAT, AND BE MERRY

Hollywood is not known for its restraint and neither are its inhabitants. Little did we know that no restraint is also the answer to beating sugar cravings.

Let's say it's a week or so before the big bash, it's that time of the month or the stress and pressure are closing in, and you must, *we mean must*, have that Snicker's bar or chocolate cupcake from *Sprinkles* in Beverly Hills. Don't beat it. Eat it! That is the philosophy of **Susan McQuillan**, R.D., author of *Breaking the Bonds of Food Addiction*. She advises, "Depriving yourself of your urge only feeds it. Give yourself permission to eat the particular sweet you crave. It will lose some of its power." You can fight the temptation to overindulge by buying only single-serving packages or taking smaller-size portions out of the bag or box.

SUPERMODEL LEAN

It's an **Elle** of a blessing when you're eternally gorgeous, long, and lean like **Elle MacPherson**, a supermodel with a super figure. The over-40 mother of two says when she wants to drop a few, she goes on an intense four-day plan where she eats only low-fat, organic meals twice a day. It's usually a medium-size breakfast and either lunch or dinner. But she skips the snacks.

BRUSH AWAY THE POUNDS

Dropping two pounds can be as easy as using a toothbrush and some Crest. **Denise Richards**'s trainer Garrett Warren advises, "When you go out, stash a toothbrush and toothpaste in your bag. Before you eat, go brush your teeth. The taste will help kill your appetite and cause you to eat less."

OLDER IS BETTER

Everyone knows it true. Take a look at **Madonna** at 27. Pleeease! Chunky, thick, and did ya see those eyebrows? Take a look at **Madonna** at 47—lean, trim, sexy, no unibrow. Or how about **Demi** at 23—big poufy hair, fleshy, a little dull. Take at look at **Demi** at 41. One word for you:

Ashton! Enough said. Yes, my darlings, older is better in many ways for today's women.

What are a few quick tips to look better at 40 than at 20? A group of actresses told us this is what works at the gym: Mix it up. Don't do the same routine every single day. Try to stay at the gym for an hour by devoting thirty minutes to cardio, twenty to strength training and ten minutes to a stretch and cool down.

SO YOU FEEL BETTER ABOUT YOURSELF!

Stop and realize that The Gap is not a torture zone. Buying jeans can be difficult for everyone and sometimes it helps to bring a friend to tell you if you look good—or if your butt looks like a building. (A good friend will tell you the truth, even if it hurts.) "I usually try on at least 20 pairs of jeans before I find something I think looks good on me. And even then I have a trustworthy friend who tells me if my butt is too big," says adorable, thin actress **Amanda Peet**.

I have two hundred pairs of jeans. I would call it a fetish or at least a collection. I buy cool jeans like True Religion, but . . . I always put on the same old pair of boy-cut Levi's.
—**Sheryl Crow**

TO CURB YOUR APPETITE (A FEW MORSELS OF WISDOM)

Here is a little trick that New York City weight-loss psychologist Stephen Gullo, Ph.D., gives to his celebrity clients who are walking the red carpet on Oscar night. Suck on a menthol-flavored throat lozenge instead of grazing on hors d'oeuvres. It will keep your mouth busy for up to a half hour, dulls sweets cravings, and is a mere fifteen calories. Of course that's lots of calories to some Hollywood starlets.

Kelly Ripa says that to buffer even the best buffet, you need to have a plan. "Never go to the buffet with a big dinner plate. Take a small dessert plate with you. Don't load up more food than what fits in the palm of your hand. That way you can eat anything, but you don't overeat."

It's the day before your big red-carpet event. Do what the stars do: Snack on watermelon between meals. It fills you up without giving you a whole lot of calories, and since it's high in fiber, it is a natural diuretic. So it curbs your appetite and cleans out your system. Translation: Bye-bye bloat!

Overheard on the Red Carpet: What A-list star is so obsessed with carb control that when he goes out to breakfast, he brings his own special carb-free bagels and a thermos of his own low-carb OJ. Then he gets his goodies out of a bag and asks the waiter to toast his bagel and find a nice glass for the low-carb OJ. Yes, this is going "out to eat," but without consuming any food from outside your home. By the way, this thin actor always leaves a very good tip for the waiters' efforts.

ALL SUGAR, NO SPICE

Those six-pack abs. The perfect pecs. Rapper/actor/hottie Usher says that he wishes he could sell "Body by Usher" in a box. "What are my beauty secrets?" he says with a whoop. "Well, I think if I led you to the well, then everybody would drink from it!" With a hearty laugh, he adds, "If I could bottle my look, I'd sell it for $100,000 a bottle." Well, we couldn't afford that tab, so it's lucky that Usher gave us a few of his diet tips for free. "I try to work out as much as I can, but I fall off the wagon and miss a day here and there. If you keep it regular with the workouts then your body will snap right back even if you miss a workout or two." He cautions that this doesn't mean couch-potato time forever. "If you let yourself go too far you won't snap back—especially if you're over 25." Usher says he's not always an eating saint. "I mean, I do eat McDonald's every now and then. I'll eat bread with a lot of butter. But I only do it once in a while and then I put myself back into my program." His favorite dieting tip? "I love chicken breasts, no bread, and I go very, very, very light on the seasonings, or use no seasonings if I'm being really good. Why? Most seasonings have some salt in them and salt retains water. The more water you can get rid of and flush from your body the better. I also drink only distilled water. It's the best for flushing the fat right out of your body."

FOOD FOR (SLIM) THOUGHT—PART ONE

Eat cherry tomatoes when your sweet tooth goes into overdrive. Why go red? These little alkaline babies tip the body's pH from acidic to neutral. This means fewer sugar cravings and a diminished appetite. The tomatoes will also get rid of yeast in the body, a substance that makes you crave sugar like crazy.

BB Extra: Broccoli and cauliflower have a similar effect.

Danish researchers have found that people who put real sugar in their coffee were *less* likely to pack on the pounds. In fact, a little real sugar in your system actually stimulates your metabolism and decreases your appetite.

FOOD FOR (EVEN SLIMMER) THOUGHT—PART TWO

Heather Graham and Jennifer Garner are nutty for almonds and eat a handful a day. It's good diet thinking because studies show that 1 ounce of almonds a day can add up to a whopping 14 percent decrease in your waist size. Almonds contain satiating monounsaturated oil, which actually blocks fat absorption. Pass the can.

HOOKED ON COLONICS

We're not saying this is the way to go, no pun intended, but stars do love their colonics. At certain detox centers in Palm Springs and Desert Hot Springs, California, you can pay up to $2,000 a week to detox like crazy. For starters, you drink tons of veggie juice, avoiding solid food, then you do a forty-minute colonic release that gets rid of impurities and aids in weight loss. After a day or two, your stomach will get very, very flat. Models go to these places for a few days before they jet off to Paris for the big fashion shows.

And now, put down your breakfast and we'll tell you how it works. Basically, the facility (and please check for one that is five-star) pumps twenty gallons of liquid into your large intestine. This is done in a treatment room with a technician who talks you through the process. Some claim it doesn't hurt (although some people say it kills) and the risks are reportedly small. If you go to a less than savory place, the same treatment can lead to an infection, especially if they use dirty water or a technician perforates the intestine. At a five-star spa, you will leave glowing. Eighty percent of colonic devotees book a return appointment.

HOW DOES SHE DO IT?

Jennifer Aniston on how she maintains near perfection in twenty words or less: "I do the elliptical and a little bit of yoga. That's basically the entire plan." Whew, and we thought it actually might be hard.

DUNCAN DOUGH-NOTS

He played the big guy in *The Green Mile* to the tune of an Oscar nomination. Chicago native Michael Clarke Duncan recently lost a mega-lot of weight with a few simple tricks "I gave up red meat last year. One night I punched up 'Is red meat bad for you?' on the computer and about two billion things came up," Duncan says. "I sat there for three hours reading. Believe me, I'm the biggest steak and burger guy, but I put down my fork." He is also a lot less cheesy these days. "I gave up cheese. I'm the type of guy who would fry some chicken and then put a slice of Kraft cheese over it to melt while the chicken was hot. Oh man! Heaven! But now it's a lot of turkey, fish, and chicken. No fried foods, either," says **Duncan**, who has never looked better.

DIVING DIVAS

An Indiana University study says competitive swimming delays visible signs of aging, including muscle-mass loss and high blood pressure by *one or two decades*. Let us repeat, *one or two decades*! So grab your suit and take a dip.

BB Extra: Remember to wet your hair and seal the cuticle before you get into that chlorinated water to reduce damage and split ends.

EURO BABES

Don't hate them because they're European, slim, and get first dibs on all the great fashion trends.

Euro women shared with us a few of their diet secrets. For instance, they slim down sipping lime blossom tea or other floral flavors. A slightly sweet herbal tea with floral extracts acts as a diuretic while preventing bloating and curbing hunger.

LOSING IT OVER BEING TOO THIN

Gilmore Girl **Alexis Bledel** is committed to setting her own rules when it comes to a career. She jumps with both high heels into a discussion about how young actresses are getting thinner and thinner to the point where they're just a big head on a stick body.

The naturally thin Bledel isn't avoiding every carb.

"When I was 14 years old and modeling, I had people say, 'You need to lose two inches on your hips.' My reply was, 'I have more jobs than I can do. I'm in high school. Why would I go to all this trouble and sacrifice for two inches on my hips?'

"You can dismiss all the pressure," she says. "Weight is not the most important thing in the world. It's totally superficial. Young women should just say no and be healthy."

BB Extra: Even the Desperate Housewives don't deny themselves in the name of being pin-thin. "We order pizza and drink wine," **Eva Longoria** says.

Overheard on the Red Carpet: What A-list star hates working out so much (just like you and me) that he went to great lengths *not* to get in shape for his new $100 million summer movie? The producers were shocked when Mr. Star showed up looking as flabby as the day they met him and cast him in the he-man action role six months before. In the meantime, these same producers had paid for, set, and scheduled a personal trainer at a hot Beverly Hills gym to make sure he was tough and buff by the first day of shooting. The trainer had reported that Mr. Big Star showed up every single day, dumped pounds, built muscle, and looked amazing. Why was he suddenly flabola? The mystery was solved when Mr. A-List confessed he had sent a look-alike to the gym every single day!

CHAPTER 11

Two-Week Countdown to Your Own Red Carpet

As long as your shoes hurt that's a sign you're at an awards show. You're at the right place.

—**Angela Bassett**

You put on an outfit and think, "Hey, I feel sexy." But I think that it's rare that you feel beautiful. I think beauty is something that you sort of recognize in other people. I never look at myself in the mirror and say, "I look really beautiful."

—Total babe **Scarlett Johansson**, who, bless her, has the same self-esteem issues as the rest of us

I'm a very lucky girl. I'm a mom with two kids. Anyone who wants to pass a fancy dress my way, I'm trying it on.

—**Reese Witherspoon**
on getting sent free frocks for awards shows

Okay, now we're in the home stretch before you step onto your own red carpet. We've detailed an intensive two-week plan to guarantee fabulousness.

First, we'll offer a few general bits of advice and then an actual weekly program to jump-start your beauty routine.

FIRST, A FEW BASIC BITS OF ADVICE . . .

Even a Note from Your Mother Won't Work with Us

Skipping one day of exercise won't trigger weight gain, but two days might. So get back on your treadmill, because you're prepping for a big night out. Why does it work this way? Well, exercise suppresses fat formation, but only for so long. So, you really do have to sweat it out on some sort of regular basis to look lean and trim. By the way, fat cells begin to store energy within one day after you stop exercising (you know who are) and this sets off a metabolic free-for-all that results in packing on the pounds, especially in the stomach.

RED CARPET 911

Hilary Swank told us that on the way to last year's Screen Actors Guild Awards, she tripped over her dress getting into the limo and ripped the hem. What could she do short of having a full breakdown? (Hint: There is no crying on the red carpet. It will make your mascara run!) "I stopped on the way to the awards and got some masking tape and just taped up the hem," Hilary says. She jokes, "Now, I'm sure people who know my background will think, 'She really is from a trailer park.'"

NAIL IT, BABY

Want your home manicure to last longer? Give your nails some pucker power. Before you polish, plunk your fingers in ½ cup of lemon juice mixed with two cups warm water and let your nails soak for about five minutes. The lemon contains alpha hydroxy acid, which will immediately make your ragged cuticles super soft without drying out your actual nails and making them crack. The acid from the lemon will also get rid of the natural oil on the surface of your nail, so your polish will go on much easier and last longer.

BB Extra: If you have some extra lemon wedges in the fridge, rub them over your winter-roughened elbows. Again, the acid will get right to work ridding you of all dead skin skills while lightening dark spots.

DOUBLE CHIN A-GO-GO

You can double your money or your fun, but it's never good to double your chinny chin chin before a big event. How can you immediately slim your face without a quick lipo treatment to your neck? A quick, temporary fix is rubbing a cellulite or eye cream that contains caffeine along your entire jawline. The caffeine will suck the water out of this puffy zone. The effect will only be noticeable for three or four hours, but that's long enough to spend your class reunion or Christmas party looking at least ten pounds slimmer.

RED CARPET SOUP

She's 40, flat-tummied, had an adorable baby, and always wears Versace low-cut, tight-fitting, revealing little numbers to the awards shows. How does she do it, you ask? Well, we asked model/actress/swimwear designer **Elizabeth Hurley**. The slim, trim Brit reveals that on most given nights she goes to bed hungry, but when she really wants to slim down for an upcoming red-carpet event she has a secret weapon: watercress soup! Liz eats up to six cups a day. It's fat free, full of vitamins, and delicious enough to serve even at a dinner party. We're guessing that you can't add the entire box of croutons!

DON'T MILK IT

Whether it's the Oscars or your block party with that one neighbor who struts around in practically nothing (we all hate her), there is one rule on dairy before the event: Don't sip anything from a cow. Nutritional consultant David Kirsch, who owns New York's Madison Square Club and whose clients include **Heidi Klum** and **Liv Tyler**, says to ban dairy from your diet on the day of the big event at the very least. David says it makes your stomach pooch out and your entire bod puffy. He also says to keep a close watch on your protein shakes to make sure they don't have a lot of bloat-inducing chemicals, additives, or soy in them, which can also make your tummy swell. More than 15.25 grams of protein in those babies might make your slinkiest of dresses feel tight.

HOLLYWOOD BEAUTY SECRETS 911

Teri Hatcher's bubbly turned trouble-y on the way to the SAG Awards in 2006. She was in the backseat of her limo in a pink chiffon Vera Wang gown sipping some Dom when her driver took a sharp right turn. The champagne tumbled all over her dress. "The chiffon suddenly turned maroon—a nightmare scenario." Knowing that she had to dry the gown quickly, Teri yelled to the driver to "blast the heat!" Teri says, "All the heat is coming out of all the vents and three of us have got my dress, holding it over the heaters in the back of the car. And it worked! It totally dried by the time I got up to the thing and I was fine!"

BEAUTIFUL TEA

Being more beautiful could be as simple as a blanket and a cup of hot tea. According to Indian Ayurvedic medicine, staying warm burns toxins. Practitioners say drinking hot fluids, eating spicy foods, and taking warm baths stave off the sick season as well. For the biggest dose of antioxidants, drink African red tea, which boasts 50 percent more of the healthy stuff (even more than green tea and black).

DIET TIPS FROM A MASTER

Jillian Hessel is a Hollywood master Pilates teacher and has clients such as Emma Thompson, Lena Olin, Cher, and Heather Graham. She says one of the biggest mistakes women make in their exercise and weight-loss regime is stopping and starting. She advises women to set realistic attainable goals and be consistent. Get a buddy, create an in-home environment for exercise, and make it a habit. Jillian also says to wear workout duds that show the body you want and the muscles you're working. No wide-leg pants with big-bellbottoms. Wear a more fitted leg so you can see your feet and positioning. Wear clothing that shows your arms so you can watch the arm movement and muscle when you are lifting or tightening. She adds that Pilates is such a great workout for women over 40 because it does not overdo those bulky muscles, but uses your core or stomach muscles and works on flexibility and strength.

IMAGE MAKER: DEAN BANOWETZ

Known as the Hollywood Hair Guy, Dean Banowetz has been "changing lives one head at a time." His client list includes Kelly Clarkson, Ryan Seacrest, Simon Cowell, Jim Brickman and others he has teased and combed out at the Golden Globes and Academy Awards. He was even featured on Oprah. Now, that's pretty heady.

You don't have to mention any names, but what are the real red-carpet 911 moments you have seen and what do you do in an emergency?
I'm always prepared. My tie is usually doubling as a place for bobby pins, which I have handed out on a regular basis for a piece of hair that is falling or if you need something to hold a pashmina together. I also have double-stick tape,

which I have used to tape in objects so nothing will pop out. I have untangled heels in dress hemlines, then applied some tape. I have sewn pockets in my socks to hold PowerBars and essentials that will bulk up pockets. It is a common feeling to be starving on the red carpet. Everyone wants to look skinny, so they are usually fasting and you never know when you may need an emergency Zone bar. I have seen hair ornaments fall out of the hair—that is why I have the duo surgical adhesive. I have helped repair seams that are pulling apart because the fabric is so fragile. I have glued earring backs on girls and I have seen so many zippers open that it is a gay man's playground! XYZPDQ (examine your zipper pretty darn quick!). I have seen food in teeth and have individual toothpicks on hand. But I think the best thing to have is some hand sanitizer because you are shaking so many hands of so many different people—fans, other celebrities, and camera crews. It's the best way to make sure you don't get sick.

Overheard on the Red Carpet: What Hollywood brain, who is truly a screen beauty (we use the brain comment in jest), once told us that the reason she looks so young is that she has been eating foods with lots of preservatives in them—and they must have preserved her face, too! By the way, those in the beauty industry we asked about this couldn't stop laughing and then told us that it doesn't exactly work that way. In fact, the less processed food you eat, the better your hair and skin.

LET THE COUNTDOWN BEGIN!
Two Weeks Before the Big Event

FOR YOUR HAIR: Top Hollywood stylists insist that two weeks before the big event, you should cut way, way, way back on all those zillions of styling products that are gunking up your hair. You don't need to be dealing with major product buildup, which will give you flathead and dull the shine in your hair.

FOR YOUR FACE: It's time for any Restylane injections, Botox, or anything that will take a short recovery process before the big event. Don't wait until the week before or you'll be fighting the clock and worrying that your swelling won't go down in time. It's also a great time to have a facial or a skin brightening like Sonya Dakar's Custom Acid Peel, which zaps zits and sun spots. Also, this is the perfect time to get your brows done by a professional who will give you the perfect arch.

FOR YOUR GLOW: Buy creams with vitamin C in them. They will lighten any hyperpigmentation on both your face and body. If you want to try a spray-on tan, now's the time to do it.

FOR YOUR BODY: It's time to clean out the impurities in your body. In other words, detox! You can get some So-Cal Cleanse, an herbal supplement that's made of fennel seed and green tea leaf extracts, which are known to kick the toxins out of your body and get rid of excess water weight.

FOR YOUR BOOTY: Virginia Madsen got ready for the Oscars by being smart about food. "I started out the day with a bigger portion of protein and carbs. Then my meals got smaller so dinner became my lightest meal. It keeps your metabolism working faster all day long."

FOR YOUR DIET: Clean out your fridge and pantry. Get rid of (or give way) all the foods that are processed or full of sugar and carbs. Hit the grocery store and load up on good proteins, fruits, and veggies. Go for organic products.

FOR YOUR SMILE: Think about teeth whitening. Don't wait for the last minute to make the appointment because sometimes it's hard to get in to see your dentist.

FOR YOUR NAILS: Run a clove of garlic over your nail beds to strengthen them. It's a little smelly, but it really does work.

MORE FOR YOUR HAIR: It's better to apply conditioner to dry hair instead of wet. Your non-waterlogged strands will soak up much more of the product. You can even let the conditioner dry on your hair and rinse it later for more shine. At the swanky Miraval spa, they put on a hair treatment to be left on overnight with strict instructions not to wash until the sun comes back up. Cindy, whose hair can frizz from someone just looking at her the wrong way, tried it and had amazing results for a week of sleek hair. She would now like to move to Miraval, but that's not possible.

One Week Before

FOR YOUR BODY: Jump into fitness. Exercise on a mini tramp. It offers the same benefits of other vigorous cardio without stressing out your knees. On the tramp, you can do jumping jacks or jump kicks. Rebounding is the fancy term for this exercise, which can burn 400 to 600 calories an hour. It also drains your lymph nodes. A home tramp burns less than $50 out of your wallet.

FOR A FLAT TUMMY: Switch from coffee to black tea. Or try drinking dandelion tea, which we see all the models buying at Whole Foods. It's a great natural diuretic.

TO FIT INTO YOUR DRESS: Do as Halle Berry does, and try upper-body twists. Sit with knees slightly bent, toes pointing up. Lean your upper body slightly back, keep hips still, and exhale as you reach across your body with your right hand as you turn your chest to the left. Inhale as you return to the center. Repeat on the left side. Do three sets of twenty reps.

FOR YOUR PEACE OF MIND: "You have to solve the whole underwear situation. I went to an awards show and I had undies on. My daughter stopped me before I left the house and said, 'Mom, I have something to tell you. *I see London. I see France. I see the lines of your underpants.*' So, off they went," says Teri Hatcher. Moral of the story: Choose your bra and undies now. It's one less thing to worry about later! And no, you can't wear the new ones today—even if everything else is in the laundry. These are special-occasion virgin undies that must stay pristine until your event.

FOR YOUR HEALTH: Michelle Stafford of *The Young and the Restless* starts her day with eight ounces of hot water mixed with a tablespoon of apple cider vinegar and the juice from half a lemon. She heard of this trick from a nutritionist who says it reduces all the toxins from your glands while giving you extra energy. A win-win situation!

FOR YOUR SANITY: Liz Hurley says to stop dissing yourself. Right now! "Never, ever point out your faults to anyone. Once you've wailed 'Just look at my hideously fat thighs,' no one will be able to look at them again without hearing your voice," she advises. So no more comments on losing those last ten pounds. Lose the low self-esteem once and for all.

FOR YOUR EYES: Eva Longoria lashes out before a big event. "Some single fake lashes on the corners of the eyes really make them pop," she says. The former tomboy who never wore makeup when she was growing up, admits, "Everything I've learned about beauty has been trial and error."

FOR YOUR FASHION CHOICE: Jennifer Lopez told us that you can't buy the same dress that your favorite Hollywood star wore to her red carpet event six months ago. "My biggest fashion tip is to dress for your body. There are all kinds of different styles because what looks good on one person simply won't look good on the next. You shouldn't feel bad about yourself. Just try on a lot of outfits." She doesn't even get too down on herself. "I'm the biggest fashion victim there is," **J.Lo** tells us. "You see things you want to wear and think will look great. Everything doesn't work on everybody. That's the best advice I can give to anybody."

FOR YOUR NEW LOOK: Consider hair extensions if you want to go long. Do it early, so you can get used to working with the new you.

FOR YOUR BODY: Do as the big stars do and get the salon treatment called Suddenly Slender. It's a mineral and electrolyte body wrap that can help you drop a dress size by draining away your water weight. Check out where at www.suddenlyslender.com.

The Weekend Before the Big Event

FOR YOUR HAIR: Get a color touch-up. It's the perfect time . . . and enough time for a fix in case your colorist messes up. (Believe us, it can happen.)

FOR YOUR HEAD: Feeling a little frazzled the days before the big party? Try to calm yourself by saying thank you to those around you who are extra helpful. It's not that Miss Manners is going to put a gold star on your bathroom mirror. It's just that studies show that people who think about the reasons they're grateful on a daily basis are happy, sleep much better, and actually work out more than people who are stingy with the praise for others in their lives.

GO SHOPPING: Buy a great eyelash curler. Our favorite is the Shu Uemura curler, which is what all the top stars and their makeup artists use each day. What you don't need to splurge on is mascara. Maybelline's Great Lash does the job just fine for under ten bucks. It also helps to purchase some triangle-shaped makeup sponges for putting your foundation on the night of your event. You can find them in most grocery stores.

Two Days Before the Shindig

FOR YOUR HAIR: Colorist Jennifer J of the Juan Juan Salon in Los Angeles, whose clients include Julia Roberts, recommends some surefire hair treatments. First, she does a deep conditioning to fill in porous spots on the hair and add a luminous glow. Then she gives her clients a clear glossing treatment, which infuses the locks with big-time shine.

FOR YOUR HANDS: Get a great manicure. If you do the mani yourself, remember to never file by going back and forth. File your nails starting in the middle and work your way to both sides to avoid splitting. You can cut the polish-drying time by dipping your nails in ice water. Or you can dry your polish by giving your nails a quick shot of nonstick cooking spray, which seals the polish and will even prevent chipping.

FOR YOUR FEET: Now for your pedi. Cut your toenails straight across and don't round them. It's also nice to give your toenails a tea tree oil treatment before you put on your polish. By the way, if you have stains from some old red polish on either your toes or your fingernails, you should soak both in water with the juice of an entire lemon. If the red still won't come out, then you can take two denture tablets and dissolve in one cup of water. Dunk, and any nails will instantly turn white.

FOR THE AHHHH FACTOR: Blame us for sending you for a full-body massage, which is soooo relaxing. If you can't afford one, then hit your tub for a good, relaxing soak.

FOR YOUR SANITY: "I try to exercise, drink water, and eat dessert," says Jessica Alba on how she gets red-carpet ready.

The Day Before

FOR YOUR BODY: Coffee and tea contribute to body odor by increasing the activity of apocrine sweat glands—special glands in the hairy parts of the body that produce strong-smelling, musky secretions. Try eliminating caffeine before a big event.

FOR YOUR HAIR: Let's say you've stripped your hair and now it looks really dull. You need to shine on, and a cheap way to do it is by using a jar of Ponds cold cream and a plastic bag. Wet your hair, put on the Ponds, and then put the plastic bag on your head. Let the concoction sink in as you do other things, which is what model Amber Valletta does when she uses this home remedy.

If you have dry hair and dry skin, you can go directly to your kitchen for a fix-a-roo. Mix up a batter of mayo, eggs, and beer and place it on your head with a shower cap over it. Let it sit for twenty minutes then wash it out. It won't smell great, but it's a better moisturizer than hot oil! You can also use flat Coke, which adds shine to dull hair. Soap star Hunter Tylo says this works every single time.

FOR YOUR LOOK: Practice covering any flaws with makeup. If you have small eyes, make them larger by applying a pale metallic color to the inner part of your eyelid. When you're doing your liner, remember to make it a little thicker on the outer corners of eyes. If you have thin lips, line them just outside your real line with a natural pencil. Use pale shades of lipstick covered with a sparkly gloss to create full lips.

FOR YOUR ZITS: Suddenly, you notice a huge zit. We repeat. Do not jump off a building. Apply an ice cube on the area for thirty seconds and then gently press a cotton pad soaked in eye drops on top of the zit for three minutes. The ice and the eye drops will cause blood vessels just beneath the skin's surface to contract, thus minimizing redness and irritation.

The Night Before

FOR YOUR HAIR: Wash your hair using a good shampoo and a volumizing conditioner. Then on the day of the event you'll have day-old hair—very shiny and much easier to style. The only exception here is if you have oily hair. Then you must wash it the day of the event. Do a test run a few days before the event to see what you'll need.

FOR YOUR FACE: If you need to pluck a few eyebrow hairs, do it right after you get out of the shower. The steam will make tweezing much easier. Remember that full brows look most natural, so don't pluck too many hairs and leave the ones above the brow alone.

FOR YOUR (YIKES) CELLULITE: Massage a half-cup of warm brewed coffee grounds onto the skin and then use a plastic wrap to trap the granules against the skin for ten minutes. You'll see the difference immediately and the effects will last up to twelve hours.

Last Few Dieting Hours Before the Big Event

FOR YOUR SANITY (AND HEALTH): Eat something. You don't want to pass out the minute you arrive. Eric Bana of *Munich* fame tells us that he eats pasta before going to the Oscars so he's not hungry the entire night.

FOR SOME PEP: Sienna Miller says one of her pre-Oscar party tricks was recharging with Emergen-C.

It's Oscar Day! (Or Class Reunion, Your Wedding, Fill in the Blank, etc)

FOR YOUR NERVOUS SYSTEM: Start early. Naomi Watts tells us, "The worst thing in the world is having to rush when you have to get ready. I like to start at the crack of dawn. That way the pressure isn't on!"

FOR YOUR SANITY: We know that this is the moment when you'll probably decide that you absolutely hate the dress you picked (or suit or pants) and that this garment makes you look at least twenty pounds heavier and is a color your mother wore in 1952 at her prom. Stop, in the name of loving yourself and your choices. It's probably too late to fret. Just remember how hard it was to make this fashion selection. Our pal **Felicity Huffman** reminds us, "Peace in the Middle East is a cakewalk compared to picking out the right outfit for a big night like the Oscars."

FOR YOUR GLAM LOOK: From our favorite makeup artist Jeanine: Layer your eye shadows, wet and dry, for staying power. Dip a Q-tip in a bit of water to moisten the shadow. (You only need a little.) Spread over entire lid (browbone to lash line), let it dry and then apply the same color to your lid with a dry Q-tip or brush. You will have shadow for hours. You can also use this wet/dry combo with your eyeliner.

FOR YOUR LASHES: Unless you're going to a swim party or a deep-sea diving bash, please put away your waterproof mascara, which should never, ever be used when going to a land-lubbers event. It will certainly clump up and even cause your lashes to droop as the hours pass. If you're worried about crying (as at a wedding) you can use water-resistant mascara, which is much thinner in consistency and won't cake.

FOR YOUR LIPS: Beyoncé Knowles, Gwyneth Paltrow, and **Kristin Davis** use Rosebud Salve, a simple $5 product that softens lips in an instant. You can find it at any beauty-supply store or in most department stores. You can also use it on your brows to keep the hairs in line.

FOR THAT NATURAL (UH-HUH) SUN-KISSED GLOW: Keep in mind that the "sun"—aka your bronzer—didn't just kiss your face. Remember to dust it lightly on your forehead, nose, cheekbones, and shoulders using a big brush. Oh, if you're actually tan from the sun (shame, shame, not good for you) then just skip the bronzer and lightly put on some tinted moisturizer.

FOR YOUR TEETH: Didn't have time to get your teeth whitened or you were scared to go to the dentist? (We know, we know.) You can do a quick trick that **Catherine Zeta-Jones** uses, which is to brush your teeth gingerly with fresh strawberries. They are a natural tooth whitener, and you can eat the rest of the berries while you get dressed, for almost zero calories.

MORE FOR YOUR SMACKER: Skip lipstick because it will smear off on everyone you kiss and be gone in sixty seconds. Instead go for a pale lip pencil and just add a shimmering gloss for the light, beautiful look that most actresses use on the red carpet.

FOR YOUR SKIN: When getting out of the shower, never dry off completely. Your moist skin will better absorb your body lotion or oil.

FOR YOUR FACE: If your skin is looking a little ruddy, choose a product with vitamin K. It heals damaged capillaries.

FOR YOUR BODY: Try a little bit of Nuxe Radiance, a golden dry oil that's made out of plant extracts and various oils. It goes on smooth and it isn't so oily that it stains your clothes. It will give you that J.Lo glow.

FOR YOUR PURSE: If your fab little evening purse is too little, just pack a lipstick to use as a quickie blusher. (Just dot each cheek with a dab of lipstick and rub.)

FOR YOUR QUEST FOR YOUTH: Try one of Oprah's favorite scents, Jo Malone's Grapefruit. Maybe you'll even get carded.

FOR YOUR GRUMBLING STOMACH: *My Name Is Earl* star Jaime Pressly insists that she does eat before going to a big event. "Last year when I went to the Golden Globes, I ate a few bites of a chocolate croissant before getting ready. No PowerBar for me. No carob. No fake chocolate. If you're going to eat chocolate then have a few bites of real chocolate. It will put you in a great mood." P.S.: Avoid fake chocolate at all costs. One word: gas.

FOR YOUR POCKETBOOK: Perhaps it's good to know that last year at the Oscars, Jennifer Garner wore around $1.5 million of borrowed Cartier diamonds, including a pair of 48-carat chandelier earrings that cost a paltry $600,000. We can't afford that kind of bling, but a few nice pieces added to reproductions can help you fake it.

FOR YOUR FACE: On the way to the event your car air-conditioning just won't kick in (damn it all to hell) and you feel that your face is getting a little bit sticky. Suddenly, you're worried that your makeup will run and you'll look sweaty when you arrive. Bring a spritz bottle, filled with bottled H_2O. Just spray your face lightly and let it air dry. One warning: Don't touch your face. Don't blot even a little or your makeup will run everywhere. The light mist of water will re-set your makeup and get rid of shine. But remember, we're talking a very fine mist.

FOR YOUR STRESS: Actress Amy Adams says she sang in the car on the way to the Oscars last year. Amy tells us that the sillier the song, the more your mood will lift. "I sang 'It Don't Mean a Thing If It Ain't Got That Swing!' " she says. "Just singing something silly made me feel so much less nervous!"

FOR YOUR INFORMATION: Marc Anthony will reveal his wife **Jennifer Lopez**'s best skin-care secret: "Happiness. It's great for your complexion," he says.

AND FINALLY: Listen to your soul sister **Mariah Carey**, who never gets nervous before she walks into a major party. "Just take a deep breath and go," Mariah says. "You can do it. You're fabulous!"

"If you let your head get too big, it will break your neck."
—Elvis Presley

CHAPTER 12

Air Kisses for All

You don't have to dumb yourself down in order to be cute.

—**Pink**

I refuse to be intimidated by aging. I refuse to be afraid or ashamed of it.

—**Salma Hayek**

If anyone invents a ray gun that undoes every face job in Beverly Hills, I want to be around when whoever pulls the trigger.
—**Cameron Diaz**, a huge believer in staying au naturel

Our final bit of advice to you is the *ultimate* Hollywood beauty secret. It's not about the lines, the wrinkles, or the need to exfoliate on a regular basis (although who really has the time). It's about finding what's lovely in your life—your family, your faith, your pets—and if you find your passion on top of that, well, those are the true ingredients to a beautiful life.

We weren't born cheerleaders, prom queens, or A-list starlets. But what we found out writing this book was that the celebrities weren't either. Just like us, they had to create themselves. We're still in the process of doing just that every single day. Hopefully, a few of the tips and tricks in this book—plus those rose petals stuffed into your La Perla bra—will help on your journey. (Note: Please take the rose petals out before you do the wash.)

Consider that even **Sarah**, **Sharon**, **Demi**, **Drew**, **Julia**, and all those **Jennifer**s have days when a pimple erupts, their eyes are puffy, and their hair goes from fabulous to frizzy.

They just have really good lighting—just like those rah-rah girls in high school. *It never ends!*

But we're not really bitter. We're just working hard to be better—and we'll keep working at it and pass along what we find on the inside.

Our final bit of advice to you is to always hold your head up high.

Because you do know that slouching puts on five pounds.

Beautifully yours,

Your new BFFs
Kym and Cindy

I used to be more of a fanatic about my body in my 20s. Now I'm in my 30s. I'm love me or leave me. It's more about spiritual connections and inner peace and being with family. Those are the really important things in life.
—**Jennifer Lopez** on living and learning

"Suddenly I realize it isn't power or recognition I want in my life. It is the wisdom and to know wisdom. I need to know beauty and the silence that dwells at the center."
—The Sabbath Life

THANK YOU

Kym and Cindy would like to thank the following:

Thank you to superagent Jan Miller of Dupree Miller and Associates for believing in us and our dreams. You turned this dream into a reality. We're very excited to continue this journey with your guidance.

Thank you to Nena Madonia, our other fabulous agent, whose energy and unwavering support and attention kept this project soaring. We consider you a part of our beauty team and a fabulous friend. In other words, Nena, you rock!

Thank you to Jennifer Holder at DMA for helping us in the early stages of this project. You were so supportive and had unbelievable faith in us.

Thank you to Hilary Redmon at Penguin for guiding this project from the beginning. Your encouragement, warmth, and excitement was so appreciated. We loved working with you and can't wait to do so again. And congratulations on your other new "project."

Thank you to all of the amazing celebrities who inspire us on a daily basis to "get it all together." A big thank-you to the makeup people and hair stylists who were so generous with their time and their information. You are true artists.

A special thank-you to recording artist extraordinaire Jim Brickman for your time, amazing talent, and for introducing two of your old friends.

Kym Douglas would also like to thank:

The most important thank-you I have is to the Lord God Almighty, from whom all good things come. I believe he held my hand through this whole process and I give all glory and honor to him.

Also to Wendy Walsh, who told me she wrote a book and her literary agent was Jan Miller. I asked for the number, she gave it to me, and the rest is history.

To my mother, father, husband, and son, your love was my strength; my Aunt Helen who told me she prayed for me to write a book and knew I would; my brother-in-law Alan Douglas, my sister-in-law Lucia, I remember being in the beach house in Malibu and you saying do it!; my best friend, Robyn Dunn, who is always supportive of me whether I win or lose. And to my friend, the always gracious Irena Medavoy, who opened her heart and her Rolodex to me and this book without blinking an eye. Without the unwavering support, encouragement, and inspiration of these family members and dear friends I could not have made this dream a reality.

To my cowriter, Cindy Pearlman, when we began this book we were two strangers who loved Starbucks coffee, beauty, and celebrities. Now that it is finished, we birthed a book together and I have a dear friend for life. Cindy, I adore you and you are beautiful!

Lastly, to my idol and a true icon, Barbara Walters, and

super producer Bill Geddes, Dusty, Jamie Hammer, Dana Goodman, and all the people at *The View*—especially the ladies of *The View*. This is the show that believed in me and started the "Hollywood Beauty Secrets" segment. It was a hit . . . the book was born. *The View*, thank you for the shot.

Beauty and Blessings,
Kym

Cindy Pearlman would also like to thank:

Thanks to Kym Douglas, an amazing partner and, more important, a good friend for life. We had so much fun writing this book together and it will be the first of many! You're a wonderful person, fantastic mom, and loyal, hardworking, fabulous, fun partner. But most important, your heart, morals, and kindness are an inspiration to me.

Thanks to Joyce Persico for your wisdom, guidance, and everlasting friendship. You're the best. You've also gone with me to Sephora so many times and have been through all my bad hairstyles! Thanks to Vickie Chachere for your two-decade friendship, wisdom, street smarts, and for the banana cake as stress relief (it works!). Thanks to Sally Kline for many phone calls and sage advice. You are one of the strongest people I know.

Thanks to John Barron, Christine Ledbetter, Avis Weathersbee, Darel Jevens, Laura Emerick, Debra Douglas, and Tom Connor at the *Chicago Sun-Times* for your many years of wonderful friendship and support.

Thanks to Gayden Wren at at the *New York Times* Syndicate.

Thanks to Richard Abate at ICM for all of his guidance and support.

Thanks to my brother and attorney, Gavin M. Pearlman, for looking out for me and for your love. Special thanks to Jill Pearlman (a fantastic mom); my nephews, Reid J. Pearlman and Cade Matthew Pearlman; Richard and Cheryl Pearlman (the best aunt and uncle in the world); Kim and Jason Pearlman; Beth Ann and Craig Pearlman.

To Jake and Cody . . . the best assistants on four legs each.

Thanks to my father, Paul Pearlman, for being my biggest supporter and for your love.

Thanks to Michael for your love, endless support, and for the dream of the future.

Beauty and Love,
Cindy